THE KIDNEYS

MONKEY PRESS takes its name from the Monkey King in 'Journey to the West', the 16th century classical novel by Wu Chengen. The story narrates the bringing of Buddhist scriptures to China; a journey which involves many misadventures and opportunities for learning. The incisive observations of Monkey are humorously contrasted with the sometimes misplaced compassion of Tripitaka, the monk under his protection. Monkey blends vision, wisdom and insight with irreverence and mischief.

CHINESE MEDICINE FROM THE CLASSICS
Essence Spirit Blood and Qi
The Seven Emotions
The Eight Extraordinary Meridians
The Way of Heaven: Neijing Suwen chapters 1 and 2
The Secret Treatise of the Spiritual Orchid
The Lung
The Kidneys
Spleen and Stomach
The Heart in Ling shu chapter 8
The Liver
Heart Master Triple Heater

AcuMedic CENTRE
101-105 CAMDEN HIGH STREET
LONDON NW1 7JN
Tel: 020 7388-6704/5783
info@acumedic.com www.acumedic.com

THE KIDNEYS

Claude Larre and Elisabeth Rochat de la Vallée

transcribed and edited by Caroline Root

MONKEY PRESS

© Monkey Press 1989   Second Edition 2001
CHINESE MEDICINE FROM THE CLASSICS:
THE KIDNEYS
Claude Larre and Elisabeth Rochat de la Vallée

ISBN 1 872468 02 0

Transcribed from a seminar organised by Peter Firebrace in London, May 1987

Text Editor: Caroline Root
Production and Design: Sandra Hill
Calligraphy: Qu Lei Lei

Printed on recycled paper by Spider Web, London

CONTENTS

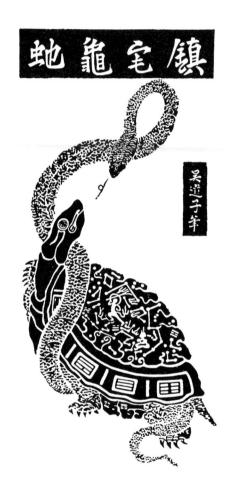

In the North there are always two animals
often the snake and the tortoise together

Su wen chapter 5

FOREWORD

The evolution of Chinese medicine in the west has been hampered by the lack of access to the original texts of the Huangdi Neijing and the illuminating commentaries that have expanded on its seminal ideas down the centuries. Without this access many students are restricted to the modern version, 'Traditional' Chinese Medicine (TCM), sometimes without the appreciation that this is definitely an edited version, since it has been subjected not only to censorship of a political regime, but also cleaned up and dressed down for scientific respectability. The irony is that real modern science is moving back to qualities, fields, interrelations, energy and the void - away from the dead-end of strict logic and over-rationality to the dynamics of interplay of heaven/earth/man. TCM has much to offer and has established a basic level of theory and practice, but it is not the whole story by any means. As Ted Kaptchuk writes in his introduction to 'The Fundamentals of Chinese Medicine' by the East Asian Medical Studies Society (published by Paradigm Press 1985):

'Idealistic, feudal, incomplete, unclear, inaccurate, metaphysical and primitive ideas that did not fit into the acceptable dialogue were omitted. Traditional Chinese Medicine was to be a neat and rational set of theories and practices.'

The present series of seminar transcripts is therefore offered as a refreshing dip, but not only into the distant past, with its world of seedling images, the coded, concentrated power of the ideogram and their skilful interweaving in the early texts, where sequence and structure themselves embody meaning. For this is not just an historical study, not some dry academic, over-intellectual appraisal of an antiquated medical system. It is vitally relevant to the present and future, not just of Chinese medicine, but of medicine as a whole. The rapidly growing systems of herbalism and homoeopathy - as well as acupuncture - are, for example, all based on an understanding of 'mutual resonance' a key concept in Chinese philosophical and medical texts. Paul Unschuld in the introduction to his translation of the Nan Jing: Classic of Difficult Issues (University of California Press 1986) has called Chinese medicine 'the medicine of systematic correspondence'. Resonance gives less implication of a fabricated system and more that of a discovery of a naturally occurring phenomenon. It is not an imposed order which has been artificially created - specific harmonics naturally resonate from a fundamental. Each homoeopathic remedy resonates with a specific symptom picture. As the text unfolds, the qi resonates - through direction, climate, element, taste, organ, body part etc. - an expression of the same quality or essence manifesting at successive levels.

The aim of this series is to deepen and enrich our

understanding of Chinese medicine. It is intended to be used alongside the more readily available material, not to replace it. The aspects covered are unfortunately often glossed over in books and courses as teachers and students hurry to reach the 'practical' side. But aren't the foundations the most important in the longer term? Look at the kidneys and *jing* in Chinese medicine underpinning the whole framework. And isn't inspiration as important as 'practicality'?

The classics are full of potent teaching, itself a catalyst for change. In this series of seminars we have been fortunate to share the knowledge of Claude Larre and Elisabeth Rochat de la Vallée, of the Ricci Institute, European School of Acupuncture (Paris). Their work on the medical classics now spans almost two decades and that work itself is founded on a deep understanding of the philosophical texts behind them - Lao zi, Zhuang zi, Lie zi, Huainan zi and others. They combine methodical scholarship with sensitive ability to weave the diverse threads of this deep and subtle subject into a coherent whole, so revealing its inherent simplicity. Their work speaks for itself and will provide a strong and reliable basis for those interested in the theory and practice of Chinese medicine.

Peter Firebrace 1989

FOREWORD TO THE SECOND EDITION

It is over ten years since the first edition of this book was published. The social, political and academic contexts in which Chinese medicine is studied and practised have changed considerably. During this time a well-trained and organized profession has emerged and there is a high level of public acceptance. A very wide range of original source material is now available in English translation, along with innumerable commentaries on and interpretations of the theory and practice of Chinese medicine.

The great pleasure and value to be found in the work reprinted here (in a re-edited version with the relevant Chinese characters inserted into the text) is that it can fulfil for us the same function as the kidneys themselves: Only that which is able to retain and hold firmly is able to stimulate that which can move outward. Only when our understanding and experience of Chinese medicine is rooted in such simple yet profound and perceptive explanations of the movement of life in a human being can we hope to circulate that wisdom and understanding outwards, to patients, to the public, to whomever is interested.

The gift to us of the work done over thirty years by Father Larre and Elisabeth Rochat de la Vallée is that it is 'authentic' in the highest sense of the word: authoritative, faithful, genuine and true. It is rooted in the classics, retained and held firmly in the classics, and possessed of a clear vision of the place of humanity within the universe. Thus grounded the authors are able to range freely in their explanations and observations never losing sight of the essential truth that all life is movement, originates in movement and without movement is dead. The kidneys, with their double nature and the constant beating of life between them perfectly embody this. There can be no higher function than that of the kidneys as 'the root of vital destiny for each particular life in its becoming', and no greater praise for a book than that it encourages and enhances this becoming.

Caroline Root 2000

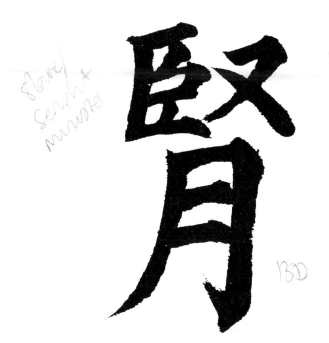

The character for the kidneys, *shen*

THE CHARACTER FOR THE KIDNEYS

Claude Larre: The character for kidneys is *shen* (腎). The part below (肉) is radical 130, flesh or part of the body, which is used in the characters for all the twelve organs except for the heart, which being master is not a part of the body, and the triple heater, which evades all the organ structures. The upper part on the left hand side is a slave (臣), but because the Chinese used to select those slaves with ability for use at court it also means a servant or a minister. It is someone who is in a prostrate and bowing position before the king (see Wieger Lesson 82E). The right hand section of the upper part (又) is the right hand itself. The hand here takes the place of the king because the one who has power is the one who is able to make gestures and to pull people along like animals, by their hand. The fact that the slave/minister and the lord are facing each other is a ritualistic position, because the lord faces south and the minister must therefore face north.

We know the difference between having power as a king, *wang* (王), as a sovereign, *jun* (君), which implies calmness and stillness, and as a master, *zhu* (主). A master is close to affairs, oversees the servants and expresses a direct power, which is not the case with the king. A king is higher than the master, because in every household there is always a master but not necessarily a king. So let us be very strict in our use of the English language in relation to the Chinese, and make a distinction between the emperor, *di* (帝), who is exalted and nearly the Emperor of Heaven, and the king, *wang* (王), who has the power to let the people feel that he has power! And the closer you come to the action, the closer you come to the master, *zhu* (主). As for the names of sovereign and prince, we may use them freely because a sovereign can be both a king and an emperor at the same time, and a prince can just imply a gentleman. In Chinese classics the Confucianist or Moralist type is referred to as *jun zi* (君 子), which indicates their quality of heart. The expression is more often used in Confucianist than in Daoist texts because the Confucianists wanted to teach social and moral attitudes and the Daoists wanted to teach authenticity.

We will be relying on the ideograms of the kidneys in order to understand their use in life's processes. Each character, for lung or kidneys or whatever, is the exact character which the Chinese want to use because there is something fundamental in the ideogram which indicates the depth of function involved. This is why we always emphasize looking at the ideograms, to impress upon you the differences between the organs and meridians according to the way they are presented in Chinese calligraphy.

Elisabeth Rochat: As Father Larre says, part of the character for kidneys is the depiction of a slave or minister in a position of respect and deference. The minister is prostrate before the master. Adding the right hand gives the idea of somebody who is able to have hold of all men. The upper half of the character gives the idea of holding something very firmly, and is the phonetic. If we add different radicals below these can indicate in which field of knowledge or reality we are. For instance, with the part of the body (肉) it becomes the kidneys, but if you add the earth radical (堅) you get the idea of something very firm and solid, something very durable. With the silk thread radical (糸) it is the idea of something important because it is urgent, and it is urgent because it is tightened and squeezed. So the meaning of this ideogram is to bind tightly. If you add the radical meaning a standing position (立) you get the idea of something upright, or to erect something vertically and firmly. With another kind of hand (手), meaning a hand in a general sense, not specifically right or left, it means to hold. Lastly, if you add the cowrie shell (貝賢), which is something very precious like money or treasure, the meaning of the whole ideogram is the sage, the wise man, the expert: a good man full of experience, virtue and knowledge.

All this is a first approach to the kidneys. But what are the kidneys in the body? The answer is that they are the same thing as the character and radicals, because they are firm, solid and durable, and they are urgent and important because bound tightly, as we saw with the silk thread radical. There are these notions of holding firmly, of being able to stand upright, and having all the wisdom which is necessary to hold the important things of life. In the human body the Kidneys are able to hold all the valuable things of life and make a firm foundation for life so that man can stand upright.

A second approach to the kidneys is through the texts of the Nei jing and Nan jing, and sometimes this can be surprising.

SU WEN CHAPTER 52

Elisabeth Rochat: In Su wen chapter 52 each *zang* (臟) is given the region or aspect which it masters, for example the heart masters the *biao* (表). From this perspective the kidneys are said to govern the *li* (裡), the intimate structure. Therefore the heart and kidneys form a couple in this relation of *biao li* (表 裡). In this context this is because the heart is a *yang zang* (陽 臟) and masters the fire which flares up and goes everywhere with an expanding movement, so the *qi* (氣) which come from the heart can reach to the *biao*.(表). In contrast the kidneys govern the *li* (裡), and govern the movement which gathers together all the elements for the internal structuring of life. The kidneys are a *yin zang* (陰 臟) and master water, which by nature is cold and condensed and has a downward movement.

Claude Larre: The *biao li* (表 裡) relationship is one aspect of the structure of man. The *biao* is not exactly the outer part of the body, it is the movement from inside towards manifestation, which is the movement natural to the heart. So when we say it is superficial or goes up to the skin we must not make this completely localized. *Biao* is just a kind of movement which displays the quality of the inner body. Similarly when we talk of the kidneys and understand that they involve everything which is for the foundation and grounding of life, we know that this is the same movement as for water and describes *li.*

Question: Could we have details of what the other *zang* (臟) govern in this context of Su wen Chapter 52?

Elisabeth Rochat: Just as the heart and kidneys form a couple, so do liver and lung. Liver gives life and birth by the left side and the lung gathers and stores by the right side. The model for this movement is the rising and setting of the sun because the ascending movement is connected with the left and the descending movement with the right. The sun rises on the left and sets on the right.

The third couple is spleen and stomach, where the spleen is the messenger and the stomach is the market place. In chapter 52, the order of presentation is first the liver and lung which relate to the daily movement of life with the rising and setting sun, then the axis of heart and kidneys with something expanding and contracting and which relates to *biao li* (表 裡), and finally spleen and stomach in the central position with the spleen as a kind of intermediary or go-between acting among all the others, and stomach like a market place through which all the requirements for nourishment and maintenance pass.

But for the kidneys the important thing to remember is the mastering of the internal structuration of the body, *li* (裡), and its centripetal and retracting downward movement.

LING SHU CHAPTER 29

Elisabeth Rochat: The quotation runs:

'With the kidneys the power of mastering is turned to the exterior (*wai* 外), by that man can hear from far away.'

The power of the kidneys, which is like the foundation of life and which holds the valuable aspects of life very firmly, also has the capacity to spread right up to the exterior and to grasp sound from far away. You know that in terms of orifices the kidneys open to the ear.

This seems a contradiction in light of the previous text. Are the kidneys mastering the movement towards the interior or to the exterior? This is just one example of the ambivalent presentation of the kidneys in all the classical Chinese medical texts.

Claude Larre: What we call an ambiguity or ambivalence here is sheer nonsense for the Chinese because they are talking about movement. When things are dead or still they are either this or that, but when things are in motion they are necessarily contradictory. They are not contradictory one to the other - but to the state when they are not moving. When things are moving they must have those two aspects. Where motion is concerned there is no ambiguity or ambivalence, that only enters when the movement stops.

Question: Is this two-way movement at all similar to that of the lung?

Elisabeth Rochat: No, it is different. Water and fire both belong to the kidneys in this context (which is different from the movements described in Su wen chapter 52). A famous commentator on chapter 29 of the Ling shu said that the kidneys are in charge of giving the beginning of the power and construction of the body, and for this reason they master the achievement of the shape of the body right up to the exterior of the body. This is the power of the essences, *jing* (精), but it is through the movement of fire.

Another thing is that in Ling shu chapter 47 when the kidneys are linked to the *fu* (府), the two *fu* related to the kidneys master the most external region of the body, the *cou li* (腠 理), which is the rhythm of life on the most superficial level of the skin. So this is an example of the deepest power spreading out to the exterior. Only that which is able to retain and hold firmly is able to stimulate that which can move outward to the most exterior part. It is only this double aspect of the kidneys which is able to make the unity of life, and we call it fire and water, *yin* (陰) and *yang* (陽).

NAN JING DIFFICULTY 36

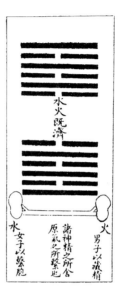

Elisabeth Rochat: Nan jing difficulty 36 presents the same idea:

'The *zang* (臟) are all single, the kidneys alone are double. Why is this? The kidneys are double: they are not both kidneys. The one on the left is the kidney; the one on the right is *ming men* (命 門), the door of individual destiny. *Ming men* is the residence of *shenjing* (神 精), spirits/essences; it is where the original *qi, yuan qi* (原 氣) is attached. There man stores the essences (sperm, *jing,* 精) and woman attaches the reproductive organs (uterus, *bao* 胞). Thus the kidneys are unique.'

In different versions of the text this last sentence varies, some say 'the kidneys are unique', and others conclude that 'the kidneys are therefore double'. But it is really the same thing.

So what does all this mean? The first statement is that all the *zang* (臟) are single: we have one heart, one lung, one spleen and one liver, so if the kidneys are double it is the manifestation of a double aspect of the power inside them. The next point is that if the kidneys are double, the double aspect of this power is that they are both kidneys and *ming men. Ming men* is the presentation of the original *qi* of the fire of life, the very spark of life by which a particular life begins.

In this text we have the presentation of the double aspect *shenjing* (神 精), spirits/essences. The spirits give the essences a good use for life, and the essences serve as a good basis for the spirits. We also have the *yuan qi* (原 氣) the original *qi*, which is on the *yang* side just as the essences are on the *yin* side. So with the kidneys we have both *yin* and *yang*. The practice of referring to them as authentic *yin* and authentic *yang* developed after the time of the Nan jing.

Something which is very old in Chinese presentations is that there is always something double in the north. For example, with the symbolic animals where the dragon relates to the east, the tiger to the west and the bird to the south, in the north there are always two animals. Often the tortoise and the snake are together. We will see this alluded to again in our explanation of Su wen chapter 5.

This distinction between left and right is quite important, but why should the left be for kidneys and the right for *ming men*?

Claude Larre: As Westerners we do not pay very much attention to right or left or north or south because direction is not of the essence for us. But if we take solar power as being connected with the origin of life, both for ourselves and for all life in the universe, then since we are able to see where the sun rises and sets, in understanding life we have to see where it starts and where it finishes. So it is no longer an arbitrary question of right and left, it is to do with assessing the natural origin of life.

Elisabeth Rochat: Nan jing difficulty 36 is really speaking of life and its transmission because in each individual's *ming men* is the starting point of their destiny, and their destiny is just the unfolding of the heavenly gift of their nature. *Ming men* is also the place from where the power to create another life from your own comes. A man stores his essences there, and in this context that means sperm. This is the same ideogram *jing* (精) in Chinese because if essences are full of life and the power of life then in man the liquid which is most full of life and its power is his sperm. For a woman *ming men* is where the reproductive organs are attached, and this is the special place of the embryo where it can develop through the double work of the transformation of essences by fire. So the sperm of a man is a liquid which is passed outside the body with a strength which compliments the power of enveloping by the woman's reproductive organs. Commentators say that as the only double *zang* in the body the kidneys are the prototype of the alliance between *yin* and *yang*.

Returning to the question of why the kidney is on the left and *ming men* on the right, another explanation could be that a rising movement can only appear from the lower part and a descending movement from the upper part. We have seen this in connected movements of heaven and earth where heaven makes its influence descend to earth and earth makes its response rise up to heaven. From this perspective *ming men* is on the right side in order to command the ascending movement, because the right side is *yin* and from the *yin* comes the fire of the *yang* which is within the *yin*. The kidneys are on the left because as the power of the water they mark the power of the *yin* within the *yang*.

Other commentators have presented this in relation to the trigrams from the Book of Change. The two trigrams are fire, *li* (離), and water, *kan* (坎), with the unbroken lines being *yang* and the broken lines being *yin*. This explanation was very fashionable at the time of the Ming Dynasty and it is very simple: fire comes first when a living being appears and it contains water or *yin* within it in the shape of the broken line. With the trigram for water it is the same in that fire is contained within the *yin* power, and this is an exact image of the two kidneys with *ming men* between them. Here *ming men* is not the right kidney but it is the *qi* and original *qi* of the fire of life which is itself between the kidneys or inside the power of the water.

One commentator on difficulty 36 of the Nan jing explained this unfolding movement of the kidneys and *ming men* by saying that the *tai ji* (太 極), the supreme ridgepole, creates the two principles which are presentations of *yin* and *yang* which then create the four symbols or images which are representations of young *yin*, young *yang*, old *yin* and old *yang*, and then these four symbols create the eight trigrams and afterwards the sixty-four hexagrams. By analogy *ming men* creates the two kidneys which in turn create the six *zang* and six *fu*, which in turn create the four limbs and the one hundred bones of the body and so on. This commentator was just explaining how the universe, starting from *tai ji* (太 極), could create everything, and how in the human body it is from fire in the kidneys and the compenetration of fire and water that all creation and construction of life appears.

NAN JING DIFFICULTY 39

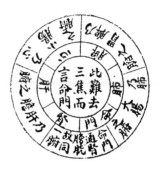

Elisabeth Rochat: This difficulty takes up the same problems again but the beginning is different because the initial question is different. The question is:

'Classical books say that there are five *fu* and six *zang,* why is this?'

The answer is very simple. Normally we say there are six *fu* and five *zang* but sometimes there are five *fu* and six *zang,* and here the basic theory is recalled. Then the answer says that when we find six *zang* it is because the kidneys are a double *zang* or have a double storing. You know that the ideogram *zang* has the meaning of to store, *cang* (藏).

Claude Larre: To hide, to keep and to store are the three

ways to understand the Chinese character *cang* (藏). We are more inclined to use store because we are usually thinking of the essences which are treasured somewhere. But other people are also right to use hide because the most inner part of life is hidden, and actually has no form. There is no difference in the Chinese between the active notion of storing and the passive notion of something being stored.

Elisabeth Rochat: You can see that the ideogram for *zang* also contains the character for slave/minister which appears in the ideogram for kidneys, and the kidneys are the supreme *zang* because they are in charge of actively and firmly keeping the essences of the five *zang* and six *fu*.

The important thing in this difficulty 39 is that when the classical text speaks of six *zang* the sixth is never *xin bao luo* (心 包 絡) or the heart governor, it is always this other side of the power of the kidneys, the power which is not water but the fire of life. We can see how in later centuries this idea gets transformed into this aspect of the fire of life at the level of the heart, like a servant of the heart. But originally the fire of life was at the level of the kidneys and it was the connection of the animation of life rising up until it reaches the heart and the heart beginning the mastering of life through the imperial fire which is natural to the heart.

Difficulty 39 continues by saying that on the right is *ming men* and on the left is the kidneys, and that *ming men* is the residence of the *jingshen* (精 神), essences/spirits, and where the man stores or thesaurizes his essences and the woman attaches her reproductive organs. The text also says that the *qi* of *ming men* is in free communication with the kidneys, and it speaks of the double storing of the kidneys, fire and water, *yin* and *yang* and so on.

Claude Larre: Would it be possible to have a comment on the fact that women are attaching and men are storing? There must be a balance between the two characters.

Elisabeth Rochat: The character for man is *cang* (藏) and for woman is *xi* (繫). I think the explanation is that the essences must be stored and kept, and so when the text speaks of a man's special essences they are something very precious and full of life and must be kept very carefully, which is *cang*. But for a woman with the intimate envelope of her uterus the problem is having a good connection with the rest of the body and with the *zang* and the blood and the *qi*, *xue xi* (血 氣), in order to permit the development of life in the embryo. So perhaps for this reason we have *xi* (繫), to attach. To attach is to be connected, and connection is important for a woman who carries an embryo.

Claude Larre: My feeling is also that it is up to the man to guard preciously the ways and means for life, and that because he has stored them diligently and carefully he is able to use them. As a counterpart to this if the woman is not able to have that which is necessary to make the essences of man prosper, then there will be no birth, no product, no child. So it seems to me that if I understand clearly what is asked of man I have a clue to understand what is asked of woman, because the same thing is asked of each, but according to their own sexual nature. The man's principle function is to keep the essences, and the woman has all the machinery which is used to make those essences into a new being. So if the woman is unable to maintain this organ in a good condition it is because the connections are not allowing that, and the attachment is not good.

Elisabeth Rochat: Because *jing* in this context relates to man, the translation can be sperm. For woman we have *bao* (包) which really means something like an intimate envelope but which we can translate as uterus or reproductive organs in this context. Men and women both have *jing* and both have *bao.* Incidentally *du mai* (督 脈), *ren mai* (任 脈) and *chong mai* (衝 脈) all originate in *bao,* which is like the first envelope of life, and protects the beginning of life. Of course for a woman, who by nature is *yin* and resembles the *yin* movement of earth, the expression of this special capacity is in the form of the uterus, which protects life for the embryo but also protects life for the woman herself in the form of essences.

LING SHU CHAPTER 2

Elisabeth Rochat: In this chapter the idea of the double storage of the kidneys is also recorded. It comes at the end of the chapter and the context is the coupling of one *zang* with one *fu*, for example the lung with the large intestines. The text reads:

'Kidneys are joined with bladder, and bladder is the *fu* of the *jin ye* (津 液).'

This is normal and the same presentation of the other *zang* and *fu* but afterwards the text continues:

'*Shao yang* (少 陽) is dependent on the kidneys. The kidneys rising, in the upper part are attached (*lian* 連) to the lung.'

Claude Larre: Why *lian* (連) and not *xi* (繫)?

Elisabeth Rochat: Because it is not a question of having a connection but of having a relationship.

Claude Larre: Why not *luo* (絡)?

Elisabeth Rochat: Because *luo* is a special network for communication.

Claude Larre: I guess that *lian* is the common word for when no special connection is seen, but there is just a normal relationship.

Elisabeth Rochat: In *lian* (連) you have the character for chariot and the character for walking. A chariot can link two different places together, carrying something from one place to another.

Claude Larre: There is no silk thread in this ideogram, as there is in *xi* or *luo*. There is no network in *lian*.

Elisabeth Rochat: It is a connection because something passes between the two places, and the connection is continuous.

Ling shu chapter 47 also sees the kidneys connected with two *fu*, again in the same context of the coupling of *zang* and *fu*. The text says:

'The kidneys are connected with the triple heater and the bladder.'

Commentaries on chapters 2 and 47 are very precise, for instance saying that the right kidney is connected with the triple heater and the left kidney is connected with the bladder. This is only understandable in the light of Nan jing difficulty 36 which we saw earlier, where the left kidney was presented with water and the kidneys themselves, and the right kidney was presented with the fire of life and *ming men*. So in Ling shu chapter 47 the triple heater is connected with *ming men* on the right, and we know from the Nan jing in particular that the triple heater can be considered like a messenger or servant of *ming men* for the distribution of original *qi*, *yuan qi* (原 氣), through the body. And the bladder is connected with the left kidney because the bladder shares the water element with the kidneys. Kidneys and bladder are also in a *biao li* (表 裡) relationship which means that they share the representation of the water element in its *yin* and *yang* aspects. We saw this in Ling shu chapter 2 as well where it said:

'Kidneys are connected with the bladder and the bladder is the *fu* of the *jin ye*.'

This is the sharing of the power of the water in this special *biao li* relationship. This text continues, as we saw, by connecting the kidneys with the lung, and this explains the double storage. This double storing of the kidneys is represented on one side by *shao yang* (少 陽), the fire which is just beginning to spread out and which is the distribution of the *qi* of life, and which is obviously the *yang* power, and on the other side is represented by the connection with the lung which is the *zang* in the upper part responsible for liquids in the body and for making them descend. In the seminar on the lung we saw that in Su wen chapter 21 the lungs are involved in the transformation and processing of the liquids in the body. The fire of the kidneys or of *ming men* is in charge of elevation of humid vapours up to the lungs through the transformations proper to the lower heater.

All commentators record this double affiliation of the kidneys to water and fire, and one famous commentator on the Nei jing, Zhang zhicong, says the two kidneys master both the water of heaven which is one and the unity, and the fire of earth, which is at the level of two. He says that this division explains the double storage of the kidneys, and that therefore *shao yang* is dependent on the kidneys and the kidneys have to rise up to have a connection with the lung. This means that by or through the kidneys, water and fire, one and two, and heaven and earth compose a unity.

Claude Larre: I would like to add something. We are in the process of evolving a new creature, a new human being, and while man and woman are still separate we are looking at the unity of this composition. So when we are talking of the origin of man we are talking of the unity of the couple, and this is the double aspect of life when life evolves from generation.

Another aspect of this numerology is that if we have heaven on the one hand and earth on the other it is sure that we should attribute the number one to heaven which gives general inspiration, and number two to earth which corresponds in a manner similar to what happens when you look in a mirror. When you look in a mirror you have the feeling of yourself and the image in the mirror, but when you are not looking in the mirror you only have the feeling of yourself. So since earth is always a replica of heaven's action it is quite normal that it should be given the number two. Adding one and two together you come to three, and in three you have the feeling of reunification because one and three are uneven numbers and one, three, five and seven show the unity of life while two, four, six and eight show more the contrast of life.

Elisabeth Rochat: So why does the commentator speak of the water of heaven and the fire of earth? I think it is his purpose to show the *yin* inside the *yang* and the *yang* inside the *yin*, which is precisely the definition of the kidneys. We know that there is water in heaven, because if not there is no rain, and without fire in the earth there is no life. It is because there is a compenetration and junction of *yin* and *yang*, and a fertile exchange between water and fire that life can continue, and the presentation of this in the body is in the kidneys because they master the the storing of the essences. The essences are always present where life is, as stated in Ling shu chapter 8 and many other places. Between life and essences there is only the difference of point of view, because essences are just the form and shape which life takes. The kidneys master the storage of essences from all the body, and they keep the special essences, which were later called the essences of anterior heaven, for the renewal of the being. The kidneys are also the source from where the *qi* can take life or the source for the *qi* of life, these are the same thing.

LING SHU CHAPTER 8

Question: Does this relate to the thirteen qualities of ourselves as described in Ling shu chapter 8?

Elisabeth Rochat: Yes, the relationship is through essences, because the essences which are stored by the kidneys are the essences which come between life, *sheng* (生), and spirits, *shen* (神), in the thirteen entities or parts. There are virtue, *de* (德), *qi* (氣), life, *sheng* (生), essences, *jing* (精) and spirits, *shen* (神), so essences appear at number four which is the number of earth.

Claude Larre: As regards number four being attributed to earth, earth takes care of what has shape and since essences are in charge of giving the exact authentic shape to an individual, earth and essences are performing a similar function, and are the same aspect of life.

Elisabeth Rochat: Another interesting thing in Ling shu chapter 8 is that in this presentation of the thirteen entities the kidneys are at the end of the spiritual aspects of the *zang* in position number five. We studied this chapter in the seminar on the heart [see The Heart in Ling Shu Chapter 8, Monkey Press 1991]. After *de, qi, sheng, jing* and *shen* come *hun* (魂), *po* (魄), *xin* (心), *yi* (意), purpose, and then *zhi* (志), will. Finally there come *si* (思), thinking, *lü* (慮), reflection and *zhi* (智), wisdom. In the middle of the five spiritual entities *(hun, po, xin, yi, zhi)* comes *xin* (心), the heart. This is not the heart as one of the five *zang,* it is the heart as the highest master of life, the dwelling place of the spirits. Amongst these spiritual aspects *zhi* (智), wisdom, which is linked with the kidneys, appears last, and the essences, *jing* (精), which are another aspect of the kidneys come before these five spiritual qualities. So we can see that the kidneys appear at the level of that which is just the formalization of life in a living being, and before the spiritual aspects of the *zang* which need essences in order to exist in an individual, and also at the end of the list of the spiritual aspects. So the kidneys appear like a bracket to enclose the highest aspects of vitality.

At the end of Ling shu chapter 8 we find the five *zang* connected with each of the special aspects of life which are under its control, such as *qi* with *mai* (脈). For example the liver stores blood, *xue* (血), and blood is the dwelling place of the *hun* (魂), and the spleen stores the nutritive aspect, *ying* (營), and this is the dwelling place of the *yi* (意). The heart stores the *mai*, which is the dwelling place of the *shen*, the spirits, and the lung stores the *qi* which is the dwelling place of the *po* (魄). And finally the kidneys store the essences, which are the dwelling place of the *zhi* (志). Wisdom Will

After the presentation of the thirteen entities there comes a description of the pathology of the emotions in six tables. The first relates to the heart, the second to the spleen, the third to liver, the fourth to lung and finally in fifth position there come the kidneys. The text says that very strong anger which cannot be stopped injures the *zhi* (志), the will. After the kidneys there is a sixth case which is not related to any of the *zang*, but which talks about fear and fright which we are unable to be free of, and which injure the essences. The important thing is that in chapter 8 of Ling shu we have six cases of pathological disorders in emotions: five are connected with the five *zang* and the last with the kidneys via the *jing*. The sixth case concerns an injury to the foundation of life through the essences, so it is not exactly the kidneys themselves, but something which is within the power of the kidneys. The very spark of life can only rise up from the essences which are both water and the element of everything which exists.

Claude Larre: When we say will, *zhi* (志), we understand will-power, and we are just using a shortened form. This should be made clear because when we talk of will in the West it is a very intellectual consideration of man's activity, but the Chinese character *zhi* is to do with what makes life within an individual emerge from the universe. They call this the will of life, so in *zhi* we must understand the roots of life where will is built and the power to organize things. This is not from an intellectual point of view, but in terms of the strength which arises from the five *zang*, and in particular from the kidneys which is where the essences reside and from where they are controlled.

Question: Why are the fifth and sixth cases of pathological disorders not related to the double aspect of the kidneys?

Elisabeth Rochat: Because essences obviously, and in this chapter textually, are connected with kidneys, and for this reason we can see that the first attack on the kidneys results in disorder in the will, but after this there is no more mention of kidneys, just of essences. This is exactly as in Ling shu chapter 47 or 2 and Nan jing difficulty 9 or 36 where there appears a doubling of each important aspect. I think that in the Chinese mind each time we reach a central important point, there is a doubling. For example, the heart has a double power in its imperial and ministerial aspects, and at the centre there is the doubling of the presentation of the exchange between heaven and earth with the rising and falling of stomach and spleen. The kidneys too are important and central because they are the beginning and they are double. The ideogram used in the Nan jing and in Ling shu chapter 2 is not the ideogram for two as in the series one, two, three, four etc, but is a special ideogram *liang* (兩), which means two as in a pair or couple. The doubling at the level of the kidneys is life as a unity but coming from a couple. The virtue of heaven and the *qi* of earth work together in order to give life. A couple is at the origin of each living being, and within each new life there is this doubling again with the kidneys which enables life to begin once more. The kidneys are the model of all coupling and the synergy inside a couple.

Question: You were talking about *shao yang* and how the triple heater carries *yang* fire energy of the kidneys. Is it the case that the gallbladder carries the *yin* water energy of the left kidney?

Elisabeth Rochat: Shao yang is connected in this context particularly with the triple heater and with the power of *ming men* according to the Nan jing, but the relationship with the gallbladder comes centuries later. The gallbladder is a special *fu* with a special connection to the essences, because as an extraordinary *fu*, the gallbladder stores essences. The gallbladder also has something to do with the uprising of life and the first appearance of life in the spring, but in the special context of Ling shu chapter 2 *shao yang* is certainly more representative of the function of the triple heater in the special link between the triple heater and *ming men* or the *yang* aspect of the power of the kidneys. The gallbladder is never connected with water.

Question: How concrete is the pathology relating to the two sides, right and left, of the kidneys?

Claude Larre: Diagnosis of the illnesses affecting the kidneys will tell you whether it is the right or left. The question is difficult to answer outside the treatment room! If a person has only one kidney, I wonder how it affects things? Do you have anything to say on that Elisabeth?

Elisabeth Rochat: It is really difficult to say because if the kidneys are the pattern for the interpenetration and synergy of *yin* and *yang* then if the so-called *yang* of the kidneys is decreasing after a time the so-called *yin* will also decrease, and if the *yin* of the kidneys decreases then you can have the phenomenon of rising *yang* which is too strong because of a lack of *yin*, and in reality the functioning of the *yang* is in disorder too. If you look at the symptoms of *yin* or *yang* deficiency in the kidneys they are quite similar: weakness, tinnitus, pain in the lumbar region and lower part, vertigo, mental confusion and problems in the sexual area. The principle is, not only for kidneys but for all vitality, that essences need *qi* in order to be carried, and *qi* needs essences in order to be released. Ling shu chapter 8 says that if the *yin* is empty then there is no more *qi* and the result of that is death. So if *yin* is decreasing then *qi* is decreasing and vitality is decreasing, and this is true of each part of the vitality of the body or the life of the universe. Within man, of course, it is the kidneys which are responsible at the highest level for this. The role of the kidneys is to manifest this interpenetration and collaboration of *yin* and *yang*.

Claude Larre: There is no answer to your question as you may see! What it would mean is that one kidney would be performing the double function which is impossible because everything exists in the crossing. The Chinese make a division between left and right and *yin* and *yang* in terms of the general constitution of man, but in a concrete case in your treatment room if someone has only one kidney there will certainly be a lowering of the power of the kidneys. I suppose the answer is that it is nearly impossible in relation to treatment to make a distinction one to another . But this is a question for practitioners and it depends on what they have observed. As for the text, the text is a presentation, and although not arbitrary it is theoretically distributing roles. In a practical case you are not helped by that.

Question: If one reads Nan jing difficulty 36, *ming men* is the residence of *shen jing.* That is not a particularly *yang* function, more a *yin* aspect, and yet very often one tends to equate *ming men* with the *yang* function, so it seems one has to consider *ming men* in relation to both aspects, *yin* and *yang.* Can you comment on that?

Elisabeth Rochat: I think in this context of the Nan jing the purpose is to present *ming men* as the origin of life, and as the origin of life it is just the junction of all that is coming from anterior heaven, *yin* and *yang,* and the kidneys are just in charge of presenting the movement of water. In this context of the Nan jing, *ming men* is really the root of the twelve meridians, the great door for expiration and inspiration, the source of the *qi* of life and so on. After this, the kidneys, which are double, represent the first division between left and right, *yin* and *yang,* fire and water. That is the perspective of the Nan jing. From another perspective which dominated in centuries afterwards, when the Chinese people spoke of kidneys they were implying the *yin* side and when they spoke of *ming men* they were implying the *yang* side. But although there is a great unity in Chinese thought, within that there are different schools, and one of these in certain epochs did say that *ming men* is the *tai ji* (太 極), the ridgepole, in each living being and that everything comes from that. That is the perspective of the Nan jing, but it is not the perspective of all Chinese texts. In modern texts *ming men* represents fire and the *yang* aspect of the kidneys, and the kidneys are the more *yin* aspect. It is a question of epochs and schools. But as far as I understand it the point of view which is common to all these currents of thought is that at this level we have something which presents the first junction of two kinds of essences, water and fire, *yin* and *yang* and so on, and that from this point all life explodes.

Question: Is it a later attribution then that *ming men* is between the kidneys?

Elisabeth Rochat: It is in the Nan jing, because when it says that the right is *ming men* and the left are the kidneys I think that it is not a physical distribution of the two masses of the kidneys, but an appropriation of the left and right. It is in difficulty 66 that we have the presentation of *ming men* as the *qi* which is beating between the two kidneys. You can see that it is a kind of sea of *qi* in the lower heater, and the *qi* is the original *qi* carrying the force of the origin. If it is the *qi* of the origin then it is also the *qi* of heaven and the authentic, and it is hidden in the depths of the back. At the level of the heart we also have the sea of *qi* in the chest, *qi* which causes the beating of the heart at the top of the trunk and in the front. So there is a vertical axis between the kidneys and heart and between the two kinds of sea of *qi*. There is also a link with the spinal marrow and cord.

Question: Is it in this text that it goes from back to front?

Elisabeth Rochat: No. But in some texts we have the notion that *ming men* is this kind of *qi* which is beating between the kidneys, and the same ideogram is used to designate the beating of the heart under the influence of the ancestral *qi* in the middle of the chest, *tan zhong* (膻 中). So it is impossible not to make the link because the same ideogram is used, but there is no text saying that, because it is not the way in which the Chinese explain themselves! They do not have an 'axis' in their vocabulary as such. They prefer left and right and beating and so on.

Claude Larre: When they say 'to spread' or 'to rise' or 'to go down' they are not talking of an axis, but the normal interpretation is of an axis!

Elisabeth Rochat: Another point is that in Nan jing difficulty 36 *ming men* is the first conjunction of our own life, and it is also through its power that we can make another life.

Question: Can you explain the ideogram *ming* (命)?

Elisabeth Rochat: The first thing is that in the upper part, two are joined as one. It is the idea of gathering. This is the upper part of another very useful ideogram *he* (合), junction, as used in the six junctions, *liu he* (六 合). Below we have the mouth on the left and the sceptre on the right. The sceptre is here for authority, because only an important person like a king can hold a sceptre. I think the mouth is here for the blowing of *qi*, and of course the mouth can also be the organ by which man gives orders, so it can symbolize the power of the master who gives orders and who is obeyed.

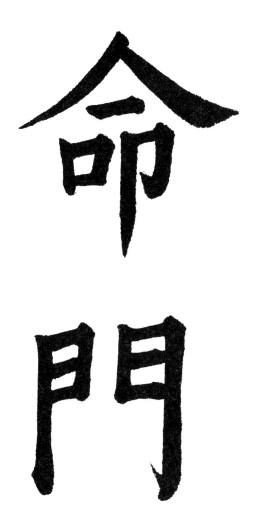

ming men

Those are the elements of the ideogram *ming*. (See Wieger Lesson 14 I). So what is the meaning? It is that I start my life through this conjunction of two other essences, or spirits, or living beings - my parents, representing the two complementary forces of the universe, *yin* and *yang*. These two essences make a new composition and I exist. I exist with my proper nature, which is the composition of elements given at the very beginning, having the ability to develop in the highest and best manner. It is a way of expressing the power and virtue of heaven in me. It is the idea that heaven for me or the destiny given to me by heaven is nothing other than the unfolding of my proper nature in the best way. This must also be according to the circumstances of life, but there is another ideogram which is often joined with *ming* - and it means all the circumstances of life and all I must do according to my nature to follow the right way, which is the way of authenticity. If I realize my nature I become authentic and I become a celestial being. It is the same with a dynasty, the so called *tian ming* (天 命), mandate of heaven, is just the same as for an individual. If a lineage has a virtue, a power which enables it to ensure the charge of emperor or warrior or king, then it has to follow that way through each of its members, generation after generation. That is the *tian ming*, heavenly mandate, for the lineage. If one day a member of the lineage is unworthy and does things which are not in the nature of the lineage and its authenticity, then the Chinese said that heaven would withdraw its mandate because there is no more power and virtue in the lineage and it no longer realizes its original and primitive nature. It is the same for man. If he becomes unable to realize his true nature he becomes unworthy and just perishes without illumination or longevity.

Claude Larre: The difficulty may arise from the fact that when someone commands us to do something we feel this is different from what we want, and that it is against our own will. Or if we do things we do not refer to any authority. But it seems that the Chinese of old thought and acted quite differently because they said that if I do something I am obeying the mandate of heaven. The difficulty is that we are unable to accept the dual aspect of heaven as both supreme power and that which makes the personal nature within myself. As long as we are unable to see that the command of heaven and the realization of our own authentic way are two faces of the same thing, it is impossible for us to make any commentary on the will of heaven or proper destiny. It is purely a question of understanding that heaven and nature are so much the same thing that the Chinese do not have two characters for them, and when they say *tian* (天), we never really know if they want to express supreme power or the true nature of things. But it is true that when they are talking of *xing* (性) as nature, they want to express a nature which is perceptible for us, because whenever the heart radical is used to form a character we know it is an actual, perceptible reality. And when they use *ming* they want to show the other aspect. *Ming* and *xing* pertain to the same highest level, but looking at *ming* I see my future which is within myself, and looking at *xing* I see the condition of my future which is my character, my temperament, my nature and all of that. So when we use Chinese characters we have to understand that they come in series, and we really have to know which one is the fountain, the source of the others. The highest source of everything is heaven, earth or man. The second layer is life, and within that we put many other characters. At the second level when we use one character there is also another opposite character to cover the area which is left uncovered. So we have *ming* and *xing*.

The consequence of this is that whenever the author of a medical book translates *tian* (天) with heaven it means that he is making a choice of saying heaven more than nature, but this does not mean that he fails to understand the idea of heaven as the individual's own nature. Conflict between people is when they oppose their natures and characters and they try to convey the idea that they are not opposing other people but are just doing what heaven has asked them to do. They forget that the other person is in the same situation. So the conflict is always in the name of heaven! But in fact it is always the opposition of what heaven is in myself, not heaven itself as such. So we come back to the question of the ego which is so important in Ling shu chapter

8, it does not say heaven is virtue but that heaven in you is virtue. That virtue is of a specific kind because you are not your neighbour, but your neighbour also has a virtue, and the word 'virtue' is common for every person. All this is clearly said in Zhuang zi chapter 2 where it alludes to one's own position and the position of everyone like oneself, who is opposing your position and those of your ranks. So you get the Tories, the Liberals, Labour, the Alliance and all that! But medically speaking the analysis is just to be able to understand the particular nature and condition of the person you are treating, which is different from the person who came just before and from the person who is in the waiting room. The good point about the Worsley school is that J.R. has been able to put the emphasis on the knowledge of the self of each patient, and around that he has built a lot of things he has drawn from the Chinese tradition. Everybody knows that his strong point is that he is able to isolate, by means of his perception, the nature of the patient, and being full of strength is able to do a very impressive treatment.

SU WEN CHAPTER 1: LIFE CYCLES

Elisabeth Rochat: In the first chapter of the Su wen the subject is celestial authenticity and how to reach this authenticity which is nature within each of us. In this chapter there is no mention of *zang* and *fu* and so on, we are just at the level where life is given and how we should behave in order to live that life fully and reach a certain longevity. Afterwards it speaks of how with this life and vitality a man is able to make another life, because I think the main characteristic of life is to give life and to make another life. Life is a continuous movement of renewal. In chapter 1 only two *zang* appear: the heart, not as just one of the five *zang* but as the dwelling place of spirits and the master of the spiritual life in each individual, and the kidneys as the source of life. The quotation says:

'Woman at seven years, the *qi* of the kidneys rise in power, the teeth are renewed, the hair grows. At two times seven years, fertility arrives, *ren mai* (任 脈) functions fully while the powerful *chong mai* (衝 脈) rises in power; the menses flow downward in their time and she has children. At three times seven years, the *qi* of the kidneys spreads out, then the wisdom teeth grow vigorously. At four times seven years, the tendons and bones are very solid, the hair reaches its greatest length, the body is powerful and strong. At five times seven years, the *mai* (脈) of the *yang ming* (陽 明) declines, the face begins to wrinkle, the hair begins to fall. At six times seven years, the three *yang mai* begin their decline above, the whole face is wrinkled, the hair begins to go white. At seven times seven years the *ren mai* is empty, the powerful *chong mai* declines progressively, fertility is exhausted; nothing passes any longer through the way of earth. The body declines, she no longer has children.

Man at eight years, the *qi* of the kidneys comes to fruition, the hair grows longer, the teeth are renewed. At two times eight years, the *qi* of the kidneys rises in power, fertility arrives, the essential *qi*, *jing qi* (精 氣), overflows up to emission; through the conjunction of *yin* and *yang* he is capable of having children. At three times eight years the *qi* of the kidneys spreads out; the tendons and bones are powerful and solid, so that the wisdom teeth grow vigorously. At four times eight years, the tendons and bones are full of vigour, the muscles and flesh are full and firm. At five times eight years, the *qi* of the kidneys declines, the hair falls out, the teeth dry out. At six times eight years, the *yang qi* declines and is exhausted above, the face withers, the hair and beard go white in places. At seven times eight years, the *qi* of the liver declines, the tendons are no longer capable of movement. At eight times eight years, fertility is exhausted, sperm, *jing* (精), is rare; the *zang* of the kidneys declines, the body reaches its end, the teeth and hair abandon it. The kidneys master the liquids, receive the essences of the five *zang* and six *fu* to store them. If the five *zang* maintain their rising power one has the power to produce emissions. But when the five *zang* are in decline tendons and bones become loose and collapse. Fertility has reached its end. So hair and beard go white, the body grows heavy, the step is not so sure, one no longer has children.'

If we look at this text carefully we can see the presence of the kidneys everywhere, both in the *qi* of the kidneys and in the exterior manifestations of the kidneys such as the teeth and the hair. In these two visible manifestations we see the double aspect of the kidneys because nothing is more soft and supple than hair and nothing is harder than teeth. The teeth are like the push towards the exterior of the same thing which internally makes the bones, and the hair is like the push to the exterior of the same thing which internally makes blood coming from essences and from the *yin* of the kidneys and so on. All the power of essences and blood arriving at the top of the head makes the hair grow, and the good state or decay of the teeth and hair are the visible signs of the rising or decline of the kidneys inside. For other *zang* there is only one exterior manifestation such as the nails for the liver or lips for the spleen, but for kidneys there are two manifestations in its dual position, the hard and the soft. For this reason teeth and hair appear continually in this text.

The text relates to the numbers seven and eight. Seven is an odd number and eight is an even number. Odd numbers are usually on the side of *yang*, of heaven and so on, and even numbers are usually on the side of *yin* and earth. In traditional Chinese thought, such as in the Book of Change, seven is the number of *shao yang* (少 陽) and eight is the number of *shao yin* (少 陰), yet we have here the very strange thing that the woman's cycles are ruled by seven and the man's cycles of vitality are ruled by eight. This is another way of making it known that the compenetration of *yin* and *yang* is necessary for life and that the kidneys are particularly involved in this conjunction because they are the model or pattern of this conjunction for our own life and the possibility for this conjunction to make another life. The kidneys represent the power of reproduction and sexuality because they are the power of the production of our own life at the beginning.

If we have a look at a woman of two times seven years and a man of two times eight years we can see this conjunction through several examples. The expression for fertility, *tian gui* (天 癸) which arrives at two times seven years for a woman is very interesting. *Tian* (天) means heaven. *Gui* (癸) shows the power of the water deep inside the earth (see Wieger Lesson 112H). It is also the tenth celestial stem which is linked with the kidneys and with the ninth stem, *ren* (壬), which we have seen previously in *ren mai* (任 脈), the conception vessel. It is not exactly the same character but it is similar. So *gui* is the water and the liquids which are full of life and which are hidden in the bosom of the earth. The coupling of these two ideograms *tian* and *gui* has the meaning of fertility for a man and a woman. It is the power to realize this conjunction of *yin* and *yang* and to make life with your own life. For a woman the expression of this meeting is through *ren mai* and *chong mai*. *Ren mai* represents the *yin* side and all that is necessary for the maintenance of the embryo, and *chong mai* in this context is the *yang* side. It is the sea of the twelve meridians. It is the impulse for life. The conjunction of the *ren mai* and the *chong mai* at the level of a woman of two times seven years makes effective this fertility, and thus she can have children. For the man it says:

'The *qi* of the kidneys rises in power, fertility arrives, essences and *qi* run out.'

In a way this is the sperm, but the sperm is just the visible aspect of the power of essences and *qi* inside the man, with essences for the liquids and *qi* for the strength and impulse. So through the conjunction of *yin* and *yang* he is capable of having children. In this context the conjunction of *yin* and *yang* is more than just sexual, it is a way of emphasizing this *yinyang* conjunction. If there is a conjunction of *yin* and *yang* you make life, your life and other life, and the kidneys make life by the conjunction of *yin* and *yang* at every level. The kidneys are mentioned here in the first position. Later on we see that all viscera are implied in sexuality and reproduction, but here in chapter 1 we are at the general level not the specific.

The last paragraph reads:

'The kidneys master the liquids, receive the essences of the five *zang* and six *fu* to store them.'

The essences of the kidneys are the essences of all viscera in the organism because the essences of the kidneys are the model or guarantee of the continuity of the individual. In another way, to make a new life it is necessary to grasp the most essential things coming from the five *zang* and six *fu*. In this sense in order to make sperm or to participate in the development of the embryo in the uterus and so on the kidneys need the purest and finest essences of the five *zang* and six *fu*.

'If the five *zang* maintain their rising in power, one has the power to produce emissions.'

The emissions are the emissions of sperm, and the power is the alliance of essences and *qi*.

'But when the five *zang* are in decline tendons and bones become loose and collapse.'

This is the untying of life, the decomposition of life.

'Fertility has reached its end.'

This happens because there is no more conjunction. Tendons and bones are an example of conjunction, and the pattern of the kidneys is responsible for the binding together of *yin* and *yang*, but if this no longer happens then tendons and bones will become loose and collapse. The *yin* has less and less to do with the *yang* and the *yang* has less and less to do with the *yin*, so finally there is separation. This happens in sexual intercourse, but also within our own body because it is the same movement.

'So hair and beard go white, the body grows heavy, the step is not so sure, one no longer has children.'

You can see that the power to have children is exactly the same movement as to have good vitality, and is linked with the kidneys.

The text of Su wen chapter 1 does not stop here because the Emperor has another quite vicious question. He says: Yes, that is alright for the normal cycles of a man and woman, but I have seen quite old men and women, over sixty four and forty nine respectively, have children, how is that possible?

Qi Bo answers:

'These people have benefited from exceptionally long life,

they have fully maintained their currents of *qi*, and they enjoyed an abundance of *qi* of the kidneys...these men can go beyond eight times eight years and these women can go beyond seven times seven years without the essences and *qi* of heaven being exhausted in them.'

We can see that some human beings have special vitality, they can have a very long life or very special strength, and this is a gift of heaven so that their nature is stronger than other individuals. If the person is able to maintain this good vitality and does not spoil it they are able to have vitality over a long time and have children during a longer period than normal. There is also a link with the kidneys via the original gift and nature, because the original gift is linked with the kidneys in the Su wen.

The Emperor also asks another question:

'Is a man of the *dao* (道), even at a very great age, able to have children or not?'

The question is that if a man is a man of the *dao* he must continuously realize in himself the conjunction of heaven and earth. But even if he transcends the numbers of heaven for human beings, or the natural laws for human beings, he is still a man. Qi Bo's answer is very simple: A man of the *dao*, even at a very advanced age is able to keep the integrity of his body and is able to keep all *yin* and *yang* together, all *hun* and *po*, all tendons and bones and all essences, *qi* and spirits. But this man, in a state of extreme longevity, is not able to have children himself, but is able to make the gift of life to children.

Claude Larre: The point is that a man, being transformed, is still a man, but being transformed there is no specific law governing him. If he is a man then he is a living man, and a living man is able to give life. So if the power to have children is natural to human kind, it is impossible that this person, who has gone beyond the limit, has not retained this power. It reminds me of Goodbye Mr Chips: at the end of the story he is sad that he never had a living son, but in his pupils he had so many sons that it compensated for the fact that his own son died. At the same time we know that the character *zi* (子) stands for disciple, master and children. For the Chinese there is not so much difference between being a master or a disciple, having children or being a child. All these are a conjunction of heaven and earth, and it is interesting to see that the first part of the first chapter of Su wen ends on this point. It may be an indication that the so-called medical books are just books which treat the human condition, and which by chance may also give treatments for this and that.

SU WEN CHAPTER 8: THE POWER TO AROUSE

'The kidneys have the charge of arousing the power, *zuo qiang* (作 強), from them come skill and ability, *ji qiao* (技 巧).'

Elisabeth Rochat: The only important thing to remember here is that the kidneys in the lower part of the trunk are in charge of arousing the power. It is the image of the double bow which is bent or stretched, and when the arrow leaves, that is the liver. The kidneys are not that which make the arrow leave, but they are the retaining power behind it. 'Retaining power' is a good expression because you know that the important function of the kidneys is to retain and keep and store. We see that in chapter 2 of Su wen for instance. But nothing is kept and retained if it is not for the upthrust, or the springing up. The power of the kidneys is the ability or possibility of producing something, an effect. Afterwards, the 'skill and the ability' are to fashion or shape something, and they are the result of charging the power.

According to some old commentaries we can see in the arousing power the specific power of the *yang* in the man during sexual intercourse, and in the skill and ability to give shape we see the specific power of the woman. But this is only one particular interpretation. The important point is that the kidneys are like the basis of vitality and the strength and uprightness of life, and it is true that for general vitality and all kinds of work if you have good bones and marrow you are strong and can work very hard. If not, and your essences are not able to give strength to your bones and marrow, you will have no strength in either bones or brain. Bones and brain need essences from the kidneys, and you need good essences if you wish to make life.

SU WEN CHAPTER 2

The three months of winter
are called closing and preserving.
Water freezes, the earth is broken up,
there is no longer any communication with the *yang*.

One goes to bed early, one gets up late,
doing everything according to the light of the sun;
exerting the will as if buried or hidden,
taking care only of oneself,
falling back on oneself, in possession of oneself.
One must avoid the cold and seek the warmth,
letting nothing flow out of the layers of the skin
through fear of losing *qi*.

This is the way that is natual to the *qi* of winter
which thus corresponds
to the maintenance and preservation of life.
To go against this current would injure the kidneys
causing weakening in spring
through insufficient contribution to the generation of life.

SU WEN CHAPTER 2: THE FOUR SEASONS

Elisabeth Rochat: Now we will look at the kidneys as the representative of the movement of water in the body, of winter, the north and so on. We start with Su wen chapter 2 because here the movement of winter is shown to be the same movement among the seasons, and of the same nature as the movement of kidneys inside the body.

The three months of winter are called to close and to store. The description of winter in this chapter is a closing in on yourself, nothing must be allowed to flow outside for fear of losing the *qi.* For example, too much sweating or sexual emission in winter would be worse than in summer because you lose essences and through them the basis for *qi.* Losing *qi* you lose warmth, and in winter you need this inner warmth of life against the cold and darkness or else you die. This was not just a metaphor at the time of writing. Therefore to go against the *qi* of winter is a behaviour not properly adapted to the circumstances. To go against the *qi* of winter means that the *shao yin* (少 陰) does not store, and the *qi* of the kidneys is powerless in the depths.

The function of the kidneys according to Su wen chapter 8 is in this strength, and if the kidneys lose this strength there is no more foundation or ground. The jumper cannot jump if there is nothing under his feet, if there is nothing for him to spring up from. This is a possible image of the relationship between kidneys and liver, or water and wood, with the rising up of life in the likeness of vegetation. Speaking in particular, if bones have no strength because the essences of the kidneys have no power there is no support for the movement of muscles.

SU WEN CHAPTER 9: THE POWER TO STORE

Elisabeth Rochat: In the same way Su wen chapter 9 speaks of the power of the kidneys in storing:

'The kidneys are the trunk in which is rooted that which controls hibernation and protects storage'.

There are four characters to consider, *zhu* (主), to master, *zhi* (蟄), to hibernate, *feng* (封), to close with a seal, and *cang* (藏), to store. The kidneys are the deep root, *ben* (本), from which all these functions are mastered in the body. The kidneys master all things in the body which are in the likeness of hibernation for animals. This is also the action of sealing up. *Feng* (封) has the earth character repeated twice and the meaning of this ideogram is to raise a mound in order to make a limit around something. It is like a border in feudal states, it is in order to protect and help something. We know that the kidneys are often likened to a barrier. In the text of Su wen chapter 61 we have the kidneys as a barrier, *guan* (關), to the stomach, because the stomach is for the introduction of food and its transformation in order to have growth and development of essences. The kidneys are the keeper of the essences and hence the barrier because these essences must never go outside the body. To hibernate, *zhi* (蟄), is also very interesting because it is the state of all the little animals before the sun of the spring. If there is no hibernation there is no consequent uprising, it is the image of the seed in the earth during winter.

'It is the residence of the essences.'

We know this already, that the kidneys are the residence of the essences of anterior and posterior heaven, of essences which are the pattern for the renewal of essences, and of all essences coming from outside. The essences coming from outside, from so-called posterior heaven, need the power of the kidneys to know how to integrate into the body.

'Its flourishing aspect, *hua* (華), is in the hair; the power of its fullness is in the bones.'

In the text it is no longer a question of the double representation inside and outside through teeth or hair with bones and marrow, it is just a question of something exterior and something interior. The hair on the exterior represents the soft supple aspect, the bones inside represent the hard aspect.

'They are the *shao yin* (少 陰) within the *yin*. They are in free communication with the *qi* of winter.'

SU WEN CHAPTER 5

The northern quadrant gives rise to cold,
cold gives rise to water,
water gives rise to the salty taste,
the salty taste gives rise to the kidneys,
the kidneys give rise to bones and marrow,
the marrow gives rise to the liver,
the kidneys master the ear.

In heaven it is cold, on earth it is water.
Among the parts of the body it is the bones,
among the *zang* it is the kidneys,
among colours it is black,
among notes it is *yu,*
among sounds it is the sigh,
among movements which react to change it is to shiver,
among orifices it is the ear,
among tastes it is salty
among the expressions of will-power it is fear.

Fear injures the kidneys,
reflective thought prevails over fear.
Cold injures the blood,
dryness prevails over cold.
The salty taste injures the blood,
sweet prevails over salty.

SU WEN CHAPTER 5: THE FIVE ELEMENT RESONANCES

Elisabeth Rochat: The character for north is *bei* (北), and we can see that it represents a position of no communication. It is to be back to back. Incidentally the ideogram for back is made up of the same character above and radical 130, the part of the body, below (背). The north is the quadrant of separation; when people are expelled or exiled they are expelled towards the north. The explanation of the north and its relationship with the back also has something to do with ritual because when man faces south (which is the ritual position for man in nature) his back is facing north and there is a communication between his back and north and his front and south. His back faces obscurity and his front faces the light.

In Su wen chapter 6 it is also the difference between life coming from the kidneys and life shining from the heart, and the difference between these two fires. Also, you turn your back in order to rebel or flee from something.

In ancient Chinese thought the north or water (because they are the same thing) was the region where the 10,000 beings withdrew to and hid. But if we return, or withdraw to something it is because it is our origin, and the 10,000 beings retire to the north because in the north, or in the water, they have the foundation of their origin. In this way we can see that the north is also the anchorage of the axis of life, and perhaps the guarantee of the supreme unity of each and every being.

There is another use of this character *bei* (北) in Chinese literature: *bei dou* (北 斗). *Dou* (斗) is a spoon or a ladle, and *bei dou*, the spoon in the north or the spoon showing the north, is the name of the constellation of the Great Bear. This constellation has the pole star within it, and in the 2nd century BC the pole star was considered to be the dwelling place of the great deity *tai yi* (太 一), the supreme unity. In the Analects Confucius makes a comparison between the right ruler of a state and this pole star:

'He who governs the people by giving good examples is like the pole star who rests immobile while all the other stars move around it.'

It was the Chinese view that the only fixed point in heaven was this pole star, and that all the constellations and other stars just moved around it. It was the fixed point of the rotation of heaven. For that reason it was the dwelling place of the great and supreme unity because it was the unification point for all the movements of the stars.

The north is also ambiguous and ambivalent because it is the separation, back to back, the place of exile and no communication, just as winter is the season of no communication. Su wen chapter 2 says that in winter heaven and earth are like strangers, *yin* and *yang* have nothing more to do with each other. But at the same time the north is also the place of returning, and of return to the origin and unity. This is very interesting because from this perspective the north is both the return to the beginning and the beginning of division and separation. In winter the soil and water are separated, the soil is hard because of the cold, and the water is also hard because it is frozen as ice; but at the same time the core of winter, according to the Book of Rites, is the moment for the mating of tigers and the period to keep seed for germination. It is the period of the tenth celestial stem, *gui* (癸), the mysterious gathering of water inside the earth ready to receive the impulse of heaven, the *yang* inside. This is like the *yang* of the kidneys or the *yang* of *ming men*, which is afterwards revealed through the *yang* of the liver and heart which are the two *yang zang*.

Of course we also have to remember that at the beginning of Zhuang zi chapter 1 the first word is *bei* (北), north. Daoists are very interested in origins and the authentic, and we can find the origin of nature and the authentic in the north and water. In Zhuang zi chapter 1 in the north there is an abyss where the great fish resides. This great fish rises up from the sea to become the great bird *peng*, which flies straight to the south. This is a good image of the power of the kidneys and heart and the rising up of life, of water and fire. So we find in this Chinese conception of the north the double power which we have in the kidneys: the separation but also the unity of the origin, the unity of life but also the seeds of diversity.

The northern quadrant gives rise to cold,

北
方
生
寒

Elisabeth Rochat: The ideogram for cold is *han* (寒), it represents a man inside straw under a roof, with the idea of freezing. The cold is the time when men huddle together under straw to make sure they do not freeze. It is exactly the movement of the north and winter and the conduct of life in winter. The north in classical Chinese books is both the place of separation and exile, and the land full of promise, and winter is both the time of closing in and a good time for sexuality and germination.

In the following quotation from the *Li Ji Yue Ling*, the Book of Rites, perhaps we can better understand how the cold is related to kidneys and bladder, and how it is linked with the *tai yang* (太 陽).

'The first month in the winter is the separation because the water becomes ice and the soil is cracked. The pheasants plunge deep into the water and become oysters. The rainbow hides and no longer appears.'

Why does the rainbow no longer appear? Because *yin* and *yang* are no longer visibly meeting and a rainbow is a manifestation of the meeting of *yin* and *yang.*

'Orders are given to the officers in these terms: the *qi* of heaven remains above and that of earth remains below. Heaven and earth no longer communicate together, the pathways of one to the other are blocked, and winter is established.'

So all the officers are ordered to cover carefully the granaries and public storehouses. The minister receives the order to visit all the granaries and private depots so that all is safely gathered in and put in a secure place. At the same time the son of heaven asks the venerable ones of heaven, the sun, the moon and the stars, that the earth should be fertile for the next year. Thus the call for fertility comes just at the beginning of winter.

'In the second month of winter the ice becomes thicker and the tigers begin coupling. Everything must be kept well closed in or else all hibernating animals would die and men would be attacked with pestilential diseases. In this month the shortest day of the year arrives. The *yin* and *yang* are struggling together because the *yang* begins to grow and the *yin* can never be as great as it is at that point. All living beings feel a movement.'

One of the commentators says that at this point all the plants prepare to give out shoots and prepare to bud. But the important point is that at the very heart of winter, at the solstice, there is a kind of intermingling of *yin* and *yang* where the first resurgence of *yang* has a particular movement which all living beings feel deep within them. If you want you can see here the power of the fire of *ming men* (命 門) and the power of the kidneys, but of course this is not in the text because that is just a particular application of a general thing in the case of the constitution of the body.

'The wise man watches over himself and refrains from acting. He comes back to his foundation; he waits to see.

'In the third month of winter the wild geese go north. The magpie starts to make its nest. The pheasant cries, the hen broods over the eggs. The son of heaven orders that a clay model of an ox should be led into the countryside to lead out the cold air. It is the moment when you prepare to till the earth.'

It is not yet the moment to actually begin tilling the soil, that comes at the beginning of spring, but they are preparing for it.

'The workers are told to join together two by two to prepare to till the earth.'

This mention of two workers can be taken to mean a couple as well, with the sexual aspect of this implied with it. Then in the first month of spring the ground will be broken and opened, and the barriers will be withdrawn so that *yang* can break out again.

If we look at the winter solstice it is like the tilting of *yin* and *yang*, a pivot, and it gives the orientation of the *qi* of life, and the first *yang* which afterwards at the beginning of spring or with the power of the gallbladder gives the direction for all the year and all the other *zang* and *fu*. I think that all the *qi* and all the expansion of *qi* move in time around this solstice of winter, just as all the stars and constellations are moving in space around the pole star.

So the cold which tightens things up is also that which will allow the springing up again of the *yang*. When the cold leaves and the earth is broken up and opened by the plough all this force and strength of the *yang* comes out and manifests itself, and these are the buds and the hibernating animals.

cold gives rise to water,

寒
生
水

Elisabeth Rochat: Water and *yin* are obviously linked. Some Chinese classics say that *yin qi* makes water. If you look carefully at this notion of water as one of the five elements in the Chinese classics you can find some strange and quite contradictory affirmations, just as was true of the kidneys in the Nei jing. For instance in the classic Chun Qiu Fan Lu the affirmation is:

'Water is the last of the five elements. It has its dwelling place in the northern quadrant and masters the *qi* of winter.'

But if you look at the Hong Fan chapter of the Book of History, which is a great presentation of the five elements, water comes in the first position. A commentator on this says water is the first of the five elements. So water is either the first or the last! I think the problem is that water is both the beginning and the end, because it is a cycle from one element to another. Of course we have to make a distinction between this and the role of the spleen and stomach as a turn-table, it is not the same movement at all. This text says:

'Water penetrates in the depths and fertilizes and dampens.'

Another thing is that water takes the shape and form of all receptacles but it does not keep any form or shape itself. And water is very sensitive to the action of warmth or cold because as a result of the cold it becomes ice and under the action of warmth it evaporates. Water is easy to touch and feel but it is also impossible to grasp, and of course, it is absolutely indispensable for life.

water gives rise to the salty taste,

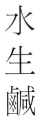

Elisabeth Rochat: Traditionally the idea was that water comes down and impregnates earth with humidity, and with this movement creates salt. Perhaps the idea is that when water penetrates the earth it becomes briny, and in this way we have the relationship between the water and salt inside the earth. And of course, we have the relationship between water and salt in the sea. Rock salt is not excluded from this idea of salt, it is even the fundamental idea which is mentioned in the commentaries, that salt comes out of the impregnation of the earth by water, as in salt marshes.

the salty taste gives rise to the kidneys,

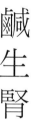

Elisabeth Rochat: The salty taste produces the kidneys because all that comes before, the north, cold, winter and the salty taste, represent the same aspect of the movement of life. The salty taste can produce kidneys because it is the result in nature of this movement of condensation and concentration and of going down into the depths. If the salty taste has this movement and power in the essences which compound it, it is able to create and recreate the power of the kidneys which are exactly the same movement inside the body. We saw with the north that it was something analogous to winter, cold and water, and water is that which goes down inside the earth with salt as the 'fruit' of that compenetration of water and earth.

Claude Larre: The difficulty for me is that there is a connection between salt and earth. One sees that there is salt mixed with soil, that I understand, but there are so many other things, and why is it more typical to have salt with water than with other substances. I noticed when I was working with Elisabeth on the text a few years ago that it was not only the ocean or the sea, and that in the footnotes they were quoting other reasons for the connection between salt and water. But I have always expected that they were wanting to expand something which was a fundamental connection between water and sea and the salt which was the first apprehension of this connection.

As regards the tastes, the names are secondary, the first thing to be considered is the movement of life which is represented. From that it is impossible to say that the reason why salt and water are associated is the sea because it would be referring to the perception on your tongue and not the movement of life. If we are consistent with the doctrine we have to find an explanation at the level at which life is moving when it is a question of water and salt.

An opposition between south and north should also be known as an opposition between bitter and salty. If north and south are constructed in opposite manners then bitter and salty must be seen in the same light. The explanation would be just what we are looking for, what sort of movement of life is it that when we are considering position we say north and south, and when considering taste we say salty or bitter? As long as we are unable to understand the movement of life which is concerned it is difficult for us to say bitter and salty are in opposition. One way to understand it is to try and trace the etymology of the characters.

The character for the salty taste is *xian* (鹹). The left part with the two strokes crossing and the four dots inside represents a rock and four grains of salt (鹵). So this is the etymological explanation of the connection of salt with the rock (see Wieger Lesson 41D). The Chinese had the same problem as we had in Europe in that salt was an highly prized condiment, and there were many places that were named after salt. Everywhere people were able to discover salt in the ground and not in the sea they were finding a rich product and were able to trade all over with it. So etymologically the connection between salt and rock is clearer.

Elisabeth Rochat: The ideogram to designate salt coming from the sea is composed of this character with something added, and it is obvious that the first salt that was known in China was rock salt.

Claude Larre: The right part of the ideogram (咸) has the

meaning to bite or to wound with the mouth (see Wieger Lesson 71). But all this does not give us what we are looking for which is the explanation of life's movement which makes the connection between the salty taste and water.

The Chinese were also very clear about the four seas, *si hai* (四 海), and the number four indicates the relationship with the four directions. We have to be very clear about this. There are wells, sources and rivers under different names. *Shui* (水) or *jiang* (江) or *he* (河) are the three most important names, along with *hai* (海) which does not mean a very big sea but is something which is not flowing and not springing up. Through the names of water we understand that the Chinese perceive water from three major points of view. One is water which springs up, the fountain or the bubbling well. Then from that water is a current becoming rivers and streams. And finally when water is neither springing nor flowing but is just there that is *hai.* If it is bigger than *hai* it is the ocean which alludes more to the horizontal expansion of water.

Elisabeth Rochat: I am struck by the thought that salty is the only taste which has a form. We can extract salt from the earth or from the sea but not in the same way that we can extract acrid or sweet or bitter or acid. We can have a salt cellar on the table but never an acrid cellar! A sugar or sweet container is quite different because of the way we obtain sugar. It is quite interesting because when water goes deeply into the earth it gives shape to the salt, and it is exactly like what happens when water, passing and repassing, leaves salt on the rocks. We can understand from that how salt can fix water because if water leaves salt behind in its flowing movement, and afterwards you put this salt back into a liquid then it will slow down the movement in the liquid because the salt retains the water.

Claude Larre: Suppose we take an amount of water from the sea and we submit the quantity of water to evaporation by fire, then what remains is the opposite of fire. Fire is the action proper to the south, so what is left has to be the opposite, and the opposite of south is north. The opposite of the pure water which is obtained through evaporation is just the salt which is left behind, so therefore the connection between water and salt is given from this quantity of water taken from the sea. That would be one explanation of the association between salt and water when it is the sea which is considered.

Now, if we take the question of rock salt we may use this process offered by Elisabeth, saying that inside the earth there are running waters, and when the water is loaded with salt some part of the salt makes a deposit and the other part remains in the water. Since the process is endless you finally get rock salt, and this rock salt is pure in as much as the constituents have been water and salt. So salty water is obtainable either in the sea or inside the earth.

the kidneys give rise to bones and marrow,

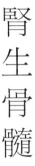

腎
生
骨
髓

Elisabeth Rochat: We know that kidneys are water, the original water and the authentic *yin*, but in between the kidneys the power of the fire of life develops, and this is the so-called authentic *yang*. We saw in Su wen chapter 8 that the kidneys have the charge of arousing the power, and during the core of winter at the time of the domination of the *yin* power, the first movement of *yang* moves the 10,000 beings. The kidneys, which are also the keeper of the essences, are also called the root of *qi*. If the power of the kidneys in the intimate structure of man is the double expression of bones and marrow I think it is because the bones represent what is hard, solid, firm and upright and the marrow represents what is supple, soft and like a thick liquid inside the bones. This is exactly like the hair and teeth on the exterior which are also a double presentation of the *yin* and *yang* of the kidneys. It is like an entire hierogamy, a conception of *yin* and *yang* at every level.

Claude Larre: One word is necessary here. Marcel Granet, who wrote about Chinese civilization and thought, and relied very much on the ancient view of things, felt that the meeting of things at a subtle level was so mysterious that the name for it had to be taken from the Greek language, and he called it hierogamy. *Hiero* means sacred and *gamy* means marriage. So when Elisabeth is speaking of hierogamy she is referring to this expression of Granet.

Elisabeth Rochat: In the couple of bones and marrow we have an example of this hierogamy. Bones and marrow are constituted from the essences and *qi* coming from the kidneys. From the quality of essences and *qi* the bones obtain their uprightness and the marrow obtains its richness for the maintenance of life and blood. There is nothing deeper than the bones and marrow in the body, and nothing more intricate and joined. Thus the marrow gives the power to the bones and the bones keep the marrow. But at the same time there is nothing more opposed: bones are hard and marrow is soft and viscous.

Claude Larre: In Chinese art when painting or doing calligraphy, the hardness or the strong aspect is seen as bone. But at the same time the fluidity has to be kept, and that quality is like marrow.

Elisabeth Rochat: In the case of the two kidneys and the fire of *ming men* the *yin* of the water of the kidneys is encircling and keeping the fire of *ming men.* In the projection of that onto the bodily structures we find the contrary, with the hard aspect of the bones surrounding the *yin* liquid aspect of the marrow. This is just one example of the continual reversals in the building of life and its maintenance.

the marrow gives rise to the liver,

髓
生
肝

Elisabeth Rochat: Why is it only the marrow and not the bones and marrow which produce the liver? I think it is because marrow represents the *yin* aspect of the kidneys and essences, and the liver is rooted in the *yin* of the kidneys, in the essences and the blood which is the liquid coming from the essences of the body. You know that the nature of the liver is *yin,* but that this nature is just the solid base for the *yang* expansion of the effect of the liver. The main function of the liver is to store the blood, and if the relationship of production between marrow and the liver is good, the water and essences of the kidneys allow the constitution of marrow, and marrow itself is necessary for the good balance of liquids in the body and the production of blood. For this reason the liver needs the support of the essences of the kidneys for its vital maintenance, and the intermediary can be the marrow. It is difficult to say whether at this time the Chinese understood the haematic function of the marrow. In commentaries some centuries later it is very well explained, so it was at least known by the 16th century and perhaps before. Anyway, if the kidneys are insufficient the blood of the liver is also insufficient, and at the same time the marrow is weaker. A lot of cases of hypertension are caused by this.

the kidneys master the ear.

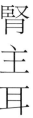

腎
主
耳

Elisabeth Rochat: The ear captures sound, and can make it penetrate into the depths. The ear can hear all sounds, it does not have a restriction of direction like the eye, but can take in from all round. So even if the eye can see almost to infinity, none the less it cannot see everything at the same time. The ear cannot hear from infinity but it hears everything that is going on all around, and it never stops working as there is no way to close your ears. Another particularity of the ear is that it is the only orifice without emission to the exterior. There are tears from the eyes, but normally there is no discharge or fluid secreted from the ear. If there is a discharge it is pathological.

We can make an analogy between the ear and the kidneys which also retain and are always working for life. It is also the nature of the kidneys to take in everything within the environment. If you remember Ling shu chapter 29, it said:

'With the kidneys the power of the mastering is turned to the exterior, by that man can hear from far away. By the good or bad state of the hearing man can know the nature, xing (性).

This is a good way to link kidneys and nature because if your kidneys are strong you have a good and strong nature, and there is some possibility of longevity. And if your hearing is in a good state and you can hear from far away, you also have a rich nature.

We know too that kidneys and ears have the same form like a bean or the moon. Another thing is that the ears are on the left and right of the head and the kidneys are on the left and right in the bottom of the trunk. In addition, on the exterior of the body the ears are the sign of longevity and wisdom. If you have very long ears, as in certain statues of the Buddha, you have a good nature, longevity and wisdom, because wisdom is also knowhow. We saw in Su wen chapter 8 that the kidneys were linked with knowhow and ability. knowhow is nothing other than wisdom, there is no wisdom without the realization of that wisdom and its efficacity. The name of Lao zi was Lao dan, and the meaning of *dan* (耽) is 'he of the long dangling ears'.

...among colours it is black,

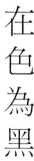

在
色
為
黑

Elisabeth Rochat: Why is it this black soot colour? The ideogram for soot black is *hei* (黑) (see Wieger Lesson 40D). Etymologically it alludes to: 'That which the fire deposits around the aperture through which the smoke escapes, soot. In the primitive Chinese huts the smoke found its way out through the window.'

It is quite strange to find the fire radical (at the bottom of the ideogram) in the character for the coloured aspect which means black, and which is linked with the north and water and so on. The fire radical represents the fire which warms the insides of the huts and it is the residual traces of this heat escaping which give the soot black colour. It is also the idea of smoking out, with the smoke rising up from the fire but no longer having the warmth or the colour.

In the pathological field we know very well that if we have a weakness in the kidneys, for example, a so-called emptiness of the *yang* of the kidneys with a tendency to get cold, this leads to stagnation, for instance in the blood. In this pathological case the black colour is an indication of the bad circulation by the blood and of the injury of the kidneys.

Claude Larre: It looks to me that, as in the case of salt and water, everything seems to hang on the idea of separation. If the heat and warmth is rising up, going to the south, then something is being withdrawn which then goes down, and this is the soot which is dark black. It is easier to understand one element if we take the opposite element and look at the process of separation between these two opposites. Man is always standing in the middle, so there is never pure red or pure anything. It is always a condition in which opposites are maintaining life, and when the kidneys are showing it is just because the heart is not having its share. The revolution of something in life is when the equilibrium of the balance is no longer kept. So in order to build a true image of the kidneys or black we have to take this combination of opposite elements and see the relationship between north and south. From this we have quite a good understanding, which is the way Zhuang zi chapter 1 is presented. It starts with the north, the ocean, the cold and the fish, and progressively it comes to the south, to the light and the bird. That is the way to look at things.

If we were looking at the east-west axis it would be that metal is just the contrary of wood, that metal is made by an accumulation of pressure on earth and that wood is made by expansion from the seeds which are contained in the earth. The difficulty in explaining things is that usually we isolate one aspect and try to say a lot about that without seeing that this aspect is never understood except by a separation within the equilibrium which stands in the middle of things. The more we talk of black or red, the less we understand what it is because during that time we forget its opposite!

among notes it is yu,

Elisabeth Rochat: The name of the fifth note is *yu* (羽). In classical texts we find that this note corresponds to water with a deep profound bass sound. Each of the five notes or vibrations are linked with something in society and its good maintenance. In books like the Historical Records, or in the *Yue Ji,* which is a special chapter on music in the Book of Rites, we find that this note *yu* represents things which are necessary for the maintenance of the people and their resources. When the vibration of this note is in disorder and the sound becomes anxious and nervous, it is a sign that your fortunes and riches are exhausted. You can obviously see all the connections with the kidneys and the body. We also find in the texts that there is a special connection between this note *yu* and the kidneys. The Historical Records say that the note *yu* moves the kidneys and puts man in harmony with the perfect wisdom, *zhi* (智), the practical kind of wisdom. If a man is able to hear the vibration of this note *yu* this means that he is able to remain in a good state and is able to practice rites, or the ritual life of society, correctly.

But what is the meaning of the ideogram? It represents the feathers of a bird. The general meaning of *yu*, when it is not specifically the fifth note, is the feathers of a bird. It can also mean the feathers that are used in dances or pantomimes. In old Chinese mythology there is a link between the north and the feather. Another thing is that when a man is able to have feathers he is a man with wings, not quite an angel, but something like that, and in Chinese a man with feathers or wings, *yu ren* (羽 人), is a way of designating an immortal, a man who has reached wisdom. It was also the way to designate Daoist priests, and there is an old Daoist expression, 'transformation by feathers', which indicates death leading to immortality. This is because feathers evoke the idea of the molting of birds, and molting is seen as a renewal of vitality. For this reason we can see that *yu* evokes the barrenness of the north and the progression to the depths but at the same time has the promise of renewal, like the opening of the new year during the winter which is the arrival of the spring and the beginning of new life. It is a question of life and death, and life through death, and these are linked with the note *yu* and with the power of the kidneys because it is always through the power of essences, *qi* and spirits that man can live and perhaps attain longevity. Remember that it is through the power of the kidneys at the bottom of the trunk that hair on the top of the head can grow. This is the meaning of this vibration in the Chinese world, it is something deep, grave and bass, and at the same time always ready for renewal.

among sounds it is the sigh,

在
聲
為
呻

Elisabeth Rochat: Shen (呻), the sigh, is of course a homophone of the ideogram for the kidneys themselves. The character is like that of *shen* (伸) meaning to spread out and extend, which has the character for man instead of the mouth as in *shen,* to sigh. This indicates that the movement occurs in the human body.

Claude Larre: Any character refers to man, it could not be otherwise, but here there is a specific extension which is heard in the sound of the sigh. This sort of sigh is an extension of the voice reflecting the structure of the kidneys. We have to pay attention to the fact that we are always speaking about something we cannot describe in itself, but from that unspeakable point there are a lot of explanations, the colour, the sound and so on, are all describing in different ways the core of this bodily element we call the kidneys. So we have to keep in mind what has been said about each of the items in order to build the following one from the preceding ones, and thus the true notion of what exists is secretly built in ourselves. We do not pay too much attention to each individual item, but rather to what is in the middle of it all. It is like when I was explaining about the east and west, north and south. It is the idea that in the middle we do not see anything, but when the separation starts then what was in the middle is shown in our mind, and we must use the emptiness and the void to understand what is explicit, and use what is explicit to come back to the void, and to nourish the knot where everything is given within our being and which must be kept in order that life goes well.

Elisabeth Rochat: We saw that a function of the kidneys is to attract and anchor the *qi* in the depths. This is very important, and if it is not fulfilled you can have asthma and other troubles with respiration. There are two ways of explaining a sigh. In normal terms it is just a sign of the good extension and rising up of the *qi* from the root of *qi*, the kidneys, to the top of the body and the mouth. In this state you are able to read aloud with a good voice and are able to give great meaning to what you are saying. In pathological terms if you have a weakness in the *qi* of the kidneys for example, the elevation and surging up of the *qi* from the bottom is difficult, and you can have a blockage. The reaction to this blockage is to sigh, with very large and long respirations in order to help the *qi* to start spreading out and rising again, therefore overcoming the blockage. So a sigh is either the manifestation of good circulation of *qi* from the bottom of the trunk or the manifestation of the desire to re-establish this good circulation.

among movements which react
to change it is to shiver,

在
變
動
為
慄

Elisabeth Rochat: We can shiver because of cold or fear, and both are linked with the kidneys. I think the shiver, *li* (慄), is always pathological because it is a reaction to a pathological attack on the *zang*, even if it is a very slight pathology. It is a reaction to an alteration towards something bad, for instance the cold. We can have an exterior cold attacking the defences of the body and this shiver is a reaction which wakes up the *yang* power of the defence. But you can also imagine a situation where there is a weakness in the *qi* of the kidneys in the kidney *yang*, and consequently the defence of all the body is weakened, because the defensive *qi*, *wei qi* (衛 氣), takes its *yang* power from the lower heater which is the *yang* of the kidneys, *ming men*. If the *yang* of the kidneys is not strong enough we do not have enough force to correctly stimulate the *qi* which should be able to oppose the penetration of the cold, and the shiver and trembling are just the manifestation of this state.

On the other hand a great fear also injures the power of the kidneys and injures its essences, which we saw in Ling shu chapter 8. As a result we have a blockage in the circulation, particularly between lower and upper heaters, the kidneys and heart and so on. Because of the attack and the injury to the essences there is a diminution of the resources available for the external zones of the body which would be used to counter perverse attacks. As a result we shiver, and we do not know if it is because of the cold or because of fear, but the two are always linked.

Claude Larre: There is another reason for this impossibility of distinguishing between cold and fear, which is that if it is cold it is dangerous. So from cold to fear there is a normal sequence. If there is just fear, there is no reason to think of cold, but since our psychological life has already given us many occasions to shiver when it is cold, when we are shivering we may recollect other occasions when we have had shivering which was due not only to cold but to fear as well. So I would give more emphasis to cold; cold would give me a feeling of fear but fear would not give the same feeling of cold. After being in a condition of coldness if you suddenly come into a room which is heated, you not only feel that it is warm but that it is pleasant and even joyful. You have come from the north to the south!

For the character *li* (栗) the Ricci dictionary reference is 3022. The first meaning given is chestnut tree, the second meaning is firm, solid, hard, compact. The fifth meaning given is the shiver either from fright or cold. So at the very beginning we have the concrete image of a tree, which is the part on the bottom of the character (木). The upper part has the meaning to fall down, especially as in the fruit of a tree. Then we also have this idea of being firm, well-rooted, which is just like the kidneys, and at the end of the explanations we come to the shivering. So once again we are talking about the same unspeakable thing; at the same time it is either a tree, a well-rooted thing, or it is a tree moving from the effect of the wind which makes the fruit fall down. If it is not a tree but the kidneys, then although you are not dead you are in a very uncomfortable position. Fear causes the same movement in yourself as the wind in the chestnut tree, and to be well-rooted does not prevent you from being shaken. Since this is said for trees and for man it proves that beyond all concrete definitions there stands something that we can only perceive in different situations and examples, and the root of the meaning is something you cannot really express.

*...among the expressions of will-power
it is fear.*

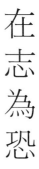

Elisabeth Rochat: Will-power, *zhi* (志), is of course, especially connected with the kidneys. In Ling shu chapter 8 we have a definition of *zhi* which says that when the *yi* (意), purpose, is conserved then you have *zhi. Zhi* is like a tension or an intensity of life, taut and fixed on a certain direction. The force of the *yi* which remains is *zhi.* In *zhi* there is the notion of something established and with a foundation. When the *zhi* remains and at the same time changes, it becomes thought. There is no mobilization with a decision in thought, rather we look at everything which can change, we calculate, combine and discuss in order to reach a project or plan. In the ideogram *zhi* we can see the power of the tension of life, and this is a specific aspect of the kidneys: tension, foundation, attention and the passage to knowhow.

The five will-powers, *wu zhi* (五 志), are the special natural living tensions which arise from each of the five *zang*. For the kidneys it is fear, *kong* (恐), for the liver it is anger, and so on. So the will-powers are not exactly specific to the kidneys but from the anchorage of the vital tensions of the kidneys there arise the five emanations according to the five *zang*. This is also the way to designate the emotions, by five and not by seven. By seven you have the seven emotions, *qi qing* (七 情), which is another thing. By five, you just have an indication of the natural emotion rising up from each *zang*, taking life or the being in a certain direction. The seven emotions are perhaps more manifest and exterior than these five will-powers which are very internal.

Claude Larre: The higher we come in numbers the more manifest is the process of life. The function of numbers is to make more and more manifest what life is, so it is quite normal that if we are operating through two we have just *yinyang*, and if we are operating with four we have the four directions, and if we are operating through five we have all the permutations and succession of the phases, and with six we have the full set of relationships between the three *yin* and the three *yang* in the unity of life. Coming to seven we have a more specific manifestation of those relationships. It is absolutely true to say that when we see at the level of seven we have vocabulary which is more explicit and manifest than when we are working with five. It is a question of tools for operating our knowledge about life as it is.

Question: When you say five emotions and five will-powers is it the same character *zhi* (志)?

Elisabeth Rochat: By five it is *zhi* (志), will-power or vital tension, by seven it is *qing* (情), emotion.

Question: What are the seven emotions?

Elisabeth Rochat: Anger, elation, obsessive thought, grief, sadness, fear and fright. What is fear? According to Su wen chapter 39: 'Fear makes *qi* go down.'

It is very important to notice that all emotions are defined by a movement of *qi*. It is not said that fear is when you have something very frightening in front of you, but rather that even if you do not have any physical cause it is the movement of *qi* going down. The explanation given afterwards in Su wen chapter 39 is that when there is fear the essences withdraw and as a result the upper heater completely closes which means that the *qi* returns below and there is a swelling in the lower heater. For this reason *qi* can no longer circulate. What this means is that fear realizes the separation of *yin* and *yang*, of the upper and lower heaters, of bottom and top and so on, because all the *yin* goes to the bottom and the *yang* is blocked in the upper part with no way for exchange or communication between them. For this reason the essences are injured by fear, and in Ling shu chapter 8 we read that:

'Prolonged fear and fright injure the essences.'

In this case when essences are injured bones are painful, we have a kind of impotence, and everything sags or collapses. And sometimes the essences descend on their own, as for example in spermatorrhoea. The explanation of this situation is that due to the separation of *yin* and *yang* there is no longer any communication between them at the level of the kidneys. Because of the fear, the essences no longer have good strength and the bones can no longer ensure their power and uprightness, and become painful. Of course *qi* and essences can no longer circulate right to the body's extremities and as a result perversities can penetrate. Also, all the movement of the body through the muscles and so on is without strength.

So, if all the *yang* is blocked in the upper part of the body there is no way to keep the essences firmly in the bottom of the trunk, and the power of the kidneys to store essences is injured, and therefore the essences sometimes descend on their own. This is the situation created by fear, and it can happen suddenly, or little by little. There is the expression 'to die of fright', and you can also say that one's hair goes white with fear, but fear can also be a situation established little by little.

Claude Larre: The character for fear, *kong* (恐), is referred to in Wieger Lesson 11F. The lower part is the heart, and the upper left means to do a work, with the upper right part supplying by pressing or knocking. So with the heart added to that underneath you have the idea of the heart pulsating and pounding as it does in fear.

Elisabeth Rochat: The ideogram for fright, *jing* (驚), shows the trembling movement, and has the character for the horse within it at the bottom (馬). It is sometimes linked with the heart and sometimes with the kidneys. It indicates a movement of surprise and fright, and can be the result of a weakness either in the spirits (connected with the heart) or the essences (linked with the kidneys). Fear is definitely a movement going towards the depths with the effect of separating, but it can be transformed into a flight from the situation. When you are afraid either you yourself move away from the situation or things move downwards in you.

...reflective thought prevails over fear.

思
勝
恐

Elisabeth Rochat: The descending movement, which is proper to the kidneys, is exaggerated as an effect of fear, and continues to the point of losing the essences. But fear also attacks the relationship between the kidneys and the heart. In Ling shu chapter 8 it says that as a result of the injury to the spirits from fear and fright you can lose possession of yourself.

Si (思), reflective thought, represents the movement of the centre or turntable, which is able to re-establish all exchanges between the upper and lower parts, to restart communication and permutation and to re-centre the individual who has lost possession of himself. We can see that reflection or thought means to see all the circumstances of a situation and the way to adapt to them. This is the best way to overcome fear.

Su wen chapter 49 says that fear is like the result of a struggle and lack of harmony between *yin* and *yang.* Su wen chapter 62 says that fear is like a result of a deficiency of blood. In both cases, *si*, reflective thought, the movement of the centre among the emotions, can re-establish good balance and good relationships between *yin* and *yang.* The spleen, which is also the centre, can actively participate in the reconstitution of the blood. In clinical practice Chinese books say you can often observe an overriding of the spleen and stomach as a result of the perverse fullness of the kidneys through fear, and the cure is to re-establish *si.* Of course thought allows you to reason and understand the situation, whereas with fear there is no reason.

Cold injures the blood,
dryness prevails over cold.

燥　寒
勝　傷
寒　血

Elisabeth Rochat: Under the effect of cold, blood will congeal, but why does dryness resolve the situation? Perhaps it is because dryness in this situation is of the same species as warmth and therefore can dominate cold. This is no longer the *ke* (克) cycle because dryness is linked with the lung and metal. But it would have been impossible to say that humidity could dominate cold as there is a great affinity between them, and they join together much more easily than they restrain each other. Here we can see that realism prevails over some sort of automatic functioning of the *ke* cycle. We also notice the implication of the blood in this particular part of the text which is devoted to the north, the kidneys and so on. Usually if we had been in some automatic run-through of the subject we would have had the bones and marrow in the place of blood, because if you look at the quotations we have taken for the other *zang* in chapter 5 then you notice that in the case of the liver it is the musculature that is attacked, for the spleen it is the flesh and for the lung it is the skin and body hair. The only other exception is for the heart because in that case it is the *qi* which is injured by warmth. So there is a couple at this level between heart and kidneys with the *qi* and blood being injured. One of the classical commentators on this chapter of the Su wen says:

'*Qi* is *yang* and blood is *yin.* Fire is *yang* and water is *yin.* The heart masters fire and that is warmth. Kidneys master water and that is cold. Thus warmth injures *qi* and cold injures blood.'

The injury comes from something that is the same type. Finally this commentator says:

'Heart and kidneys are the masters and rulers of water and fire, *yin* and *yang*, and this is the reason why the presentation is different from the other *zang.*'

So we can see that this text is never just the application of some kind of data table, there are always exceptions and rule breakings, because that is how life works!

Claude Larre: Maybe it is the verticality of the relationship between north and south and heart and kidneys which makes the relationship so immediate because it is not the same thing as going from one *zang* to another according to a certain order, or the cycles of *sheng* (生) and *ke* (克). Going up and down might be like the structure of life which is to receive the influx of heaven through earth and to rise up. It would be quite normal that the relationship of heart and kidneys would have a privileged position in the presentation. The same might be said of the middle. It is different when you want to go from north to east, for example. So when Elisabeth says there is an exception it may just be that something more simple is going on.

The salty taste injures the blood,
sweet prevails over salty.

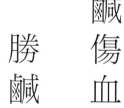

Elisabeth Rochat: The salty taste has the characteristic of softening, and too much injures the blood and leads to a dryness. We know very well that if you eat too much of the salty taste it makes you thirsty, this is said in Ling shu chapter 63, and is a sign of the diminution of bodily liquids. According to Ling shu chapter 63 the salty taste goes to the blood by affinity, and as a result there is stagnation and congealing of the blood. The same thing happens to the juices of the stomach. But the sweet taste has the ability to increase the liquids in the body, particularly the *jin* (津), and the clear liquids produced by the spleen. By this means we can bring a good humidification to the network of animation carrying the blood and re-establish the liquid flux and movement of circulation, thus removing dryness and thirst. This is the *ke* (克) cycle once again.

CONCLUSION

Elisabeth Rochat: The kidneys, themselves the basis of life, arouse the power of life in each *zang* through the fire which is in them or between them.

Through their care and responsibility for the essences, they also provide for the stability of each *zang*. They are responsible for the water which rises to balance the fire of the heart. They are the point of departure for the humid vapours that exist in the lung, permeating its numerous alveoli. They supply the basis and the model for the storage of blood in the liver and they are, with the spleen, the guarantors responsible for the right proportion of humidity and liquids in the body. A weakening of this domain of the power of the kidneys will therefore be reflected in diverse symptoms affecting either more this or more that *zang*, according to each case.

One must also understand the function of the kidneys at every level of activity of the organism: mastering water, keeping the liquids in the right proportion, retaining and drawing downwards, all the while guarding against the exaggeration of this movement that is so natural to them.

The Su wen in chapter 81 discusses the uncontrolled flow of tears and mucus through an attack on the will, *zhi* (志). It explains how the kidneys, representing the water of which the will is the most profound emanation and support, are responsible for the proper control of liquids and of water everywhere in the organism.

'The ancestor of water (*shui zong* 水 宗), is water in accumulation (*ji shui* 積 水). Water in accumulation is the supreme *yin*. The supreme *yin* is the essences of the kidneys. When the water of the ancestral essences, (*zong jing* 宗 精), cannot escape then the essences are retained with firmness.'

The ancestor of water (*shui zong* 水 宗), is the principle of gathering together, of the unified command of all that concerns water in the living being. Water in accumulation (*ji shui* 積 水) is water with all its virtue, which is continually renewed and accumulated. The water of the ancestral essences (*zong jing* 宗 精) are the essences gathered together under a unified command, by a directive principle recognized and respected by all. Therefore when the kidneys, or the will, are attacked and weakened, the firm control of the essences will be disturbed: leading to the essences escaping in the form of the *ye* (液) liquids. This is the reason why the Ling shu chapter 28 recommends tonifying the *shao yin* (少 陰) of the leg (kidney meridian) when saliva flows from the mouth.

Tears can leave the eyes and mucus can leave the nose from the effect of sadness and from the heart being shaken, and saliva can run from the mouth because the spleen is injured, but this does not preclude these liquids escaping the control of the kidneys for other reasons. Therefore the will (*zhi* 志) must keep guard everywhere and ensure the sealing and closing up of what is essential for vitality.

This same force of retaining and of will, refers us back to the *yang* aspect of the kidneys. This is a perpetual return and an endless cycle in which the kidneys, through their double aspect, can appear as the privileged returning point, and the coupling of *yin* and *yang*, whose effects are so well expressed in Su wen chapter 3:

The *yin* is that which in storing the essences allows springing up, and the *yang* is that which in ensuring defence on the exterior, keeps everything in good order.'

APPENDIX

APPENDIX

NOTES FROM THE ORIGINAL SEMINAR

EXTRACT FROM THE NEIJING JINGYI

'There is one kidney on the left and one kidney on the right (which includes *ming men*). The kidney meridian has a *luo* (絡) relationship with the bladder. It also has a *biao li* (internal/external) relationship with the bladder.

In parts of the body, the kidneys are linked with the bones and open their orifice at the ear. Their functions are to store the essences, *cang jing* (藏 精), to be the source of reproduction and growth, to master the bones and marrow, to master the five *ye, wu ye* (五 液) (the five kinds of interstitial fluids), so as to maintain the balance and metabolism of the fluids inside the body and to give their full extension to the faculty of hearing through the *qi* of the kidneys. But the most important physiological role of the kidneys is to be the root of vital destiny for each particular life in its becoming, *sheng ming* (生 命). It is because of this that the kidneys are called by the ancients the trunk in which anterior heaven is rooted, *xian tian zhi ben* (先 天 之 本).'

FUNCTIONS OF THE KIDNEYS

1. *The kidneys store the essences.*

The essences, *jing* (精), are the fundamental substance of vitality in each particular life. There are the sexual essences of both the male and female which are able to combine to make a new life. There are also essences which are produced through the transformation of solid and liquid food and which are the nourishing substance for the maintenance of life.

The first are called essences of anterior heaven, *xian tian zhi jing* (先 天 之 精). The second are called essences of posterior heaven, *hou tian zhi jing* (後 天 之 精). Both are stored in the kidneys. The essences of anterior heaven are received from the father and mother. From the beginning of embryonic life they continue without interruption until old age and only death brings them to an end. They continuously set in motion and distribute the vital force, and unceasingly produce and promote growth. But the formation of the essences of anterior heaven, especially after birth, rely for their maintenance on the essences that result from the transformation of solid and liquid food. It is the solid and liquid food which, through transformation, give the essences. But these essences of posterior heaven must rely on the abilities of the moving power of the essences of anterior heaven. The two are inextricably linked and connected.

To store the essences is the most important function of the kidneys. It is undeniable that the proper growth and development of the body, as well as a healthy constitution, are related to the kidneys' role of storing the essences.

When essences stored in the kidneys are sufficient, then the *qi* of the kidneys rises in power, *sheng* (盛). But when the essences stored in the kidneys are insufficient, then the *qi* of the kidneys declines, *shuai* (衰). The rising power and decline of the *qi* of the kidneys are thus closely related to the whole development of the body, as is seen in Su wen chapter 1.

2. *The kidneys master the marrow and the bones. Their flourishing aspect is in the hair.*

The kidneys have the capacity to produce (*sheng* 生) the marrow. The marrow is stored in the hollows of the bones to plenify and nourish them. This kidney function of producing the marrow is part of their function of storing the essences.

What nourishes and maintains the hair comes from the

blood. For this reason the hair is called 'the excess of blood'. But the mechanics of producing the hair derive originally from the *qi* of the kidneys. Because of this the hair is the flourishing aspect of the kidneys manifesting on the exterior. The process of hair growth reflects the rising in power or decline of the kidneys. For example, when one is in the prime of life, the *qi* of the kidneys is full and rises in power and the hair is shiny and glossy. But in old age, as the *qi* of the kidneys progressively declines, the hair whitens and falls out easily. One can observe whether the hair is in a healthy state or dried out so as to gauge the rising in power or decline of the *qi* of the kidneys.

3. *The kidneys have charge of arousing the power. Skill and ability stem from them.*

That the kidneys master that which arouses the power, and that skill and ability result from this is an effect of the kidney functions of storing essences, producing marrow and governing the bones.

Thus, when the kidney *qi* thrives and rises in power, the essences are in fullness and the marrow is sufficient, which means not only that the *jing shen* (精 神) is prosperous and healthy and that one is agile, alert and lively, but also that the muscles and bones are full of strength and power and that movement is vigorous.

If on the contrary the kidneys are in a bad state, the essences empty and the marrow insufficient, then it often happens that there are sharp pains in the lumbar region and back, that the bones are weak and without strength, that the *jing shen* (精 神) are tired and weary, and that there is vertigo and loss of memory.

4. *The kidneys master the liquids.*

The kidneys have the primary role in the metabolism of body fluids. If the kidneys are disordered, effective action on the fluids is lost and then one cannot maintain the balance of the body's fluid metabolism.

The liquids enter the stomach, then from the spleen they rise and are transported to the lung. The *qi* of the lung has a descending action and the liquids flow downwards and return to the kidneys. This is the general process of raising and lowering those liquids inside the body which come from outside.

The liquids can be clear, *qing* (清) and unclear, *zhuo* (濁). The clear rises and ascends; the unclear descends and is lowered. Within the clear there is the unclear; within the unclear there is the clear.

The liquids that rise up to the lung are the clear *qi*. The clear within the clear is that which, from the lung, is transported right out to the skin and body hair.

The unclear within the clear is that which, from the passages, canals and irrigations of the three heaters, descends and reaches the kidneys. The liquids that return to the kidneys are unclear.

The unclear which is within the unclear is that which is excreted to the outside from the bladder.

The clear which is within the unclear is that which passes once more through the transformation of *qi, qi hua* (氣 化), of the three heaters and rises up to the lung. These liquids descend once again from the lung where they undergo transformation down to the kidneys.

It is like an continuous circulation, an endless circle to maintain the balance of the body fluids.

EXTRACT FROM THE ZHONG YIJI QULI LUN

'The function of the bladder is essentially to collect and excrete the urine. After the liquids have passed through the separation process of sifting the clear and unclear in the kidneys, the surplus and waste flow into the bladder which collects them. They build up there to a certain quantity and go out to the exterior via the excretory apparatus.

This function of the bladder is called the transformation of the *qi*, *qi hua* (氣 化).

The transformation of the *qi* natural to the bladder is closely related to the capacity of opening and closing of the kidney *qi*. When this function of opening and closing of the kidneys loses its regulation then loss of regulation in the function of transformation of the *qi* of the bladder can appear.

The pathology of the bladder - anuria, polyuria, incontinence, dysuria, painful micturation and so on - leaving aside of course the origin of these disorders in the bladder itself, has much to do with the disorders of the kidneys.

The kidney is the *zang* which depends upon the internal (*li* 裡), the bladder is the *fu* that depends on the external (*biao* 表), their meridians have reciprocal relations of connection, *luo* (絡), and dependence, *shu* (屬).

There is a relationship between the excretory role of the bladder and the rising in power or decline in *qi* of the kidneys. When the *qi* of the kidneys is in perfect fullness, the urine is excreted at the right time by the bladder; it undergoes the function of transformation by the *qi* of the bladder and is excreted.

If the kidney *qi* is empty and cannot retain firmly, then there is polyuria, urinary incontinence and loss of control over micturation. The kidneys being empty, the transformation of *qi* is not carried out and then there is anuria and troubles with the flow of urine.'

To sum up, in traditional Chinese medicine, the kidneys encompass the urinary and reproductive functions, the internal secretions and the central nervous system of modern medicine, with all their attendant pathology. The bladder in traditional Chinese medicine is practically the same as that of modern medicine.

KIDNEY PATHOLOGY

PRINCIPAL CAUSES OF DISEASE

1. The six perverse influences, *liu yin* (六 淫)

Wind, *feng* (風), which can cause diseases of 'wind and water', *feng shui* (風 水).

Cold, *han* (寒), is the *yin* perverse influence par excellence and has the same nature as water and the kidneys.

The other perverse influences, fire (*huo* 火), dampness (*shi* 濕), and dryness (*zao* 燥), can also injure the kidneys, either directly or indirectly.

2. The seven emotions, *qi qing* (七 情)

Anger (*nu* 怒) empties the *yin* (an example of the 'son', the liver/wood, stealing the *qi* from the 'mother', the kidneys/water).

Fear (*kong* 恐) leads to unrestrained collapse.

Starting with fright (*jing* 驚) leads to a separation of the *yin* and the *yang.*

3. Other causes

Worries and excessive tiredness weakens the kidney *qi.* Sexual excess injures the essences/*qi* (*jing qi* 精 氣) of the kidneys.

PRINCIPAL SYMPTOMS

1. Sharp pains and softening of the lumbar area and the knees, *yao xi suan ruan* (腰 膝 酸 軟), lumbago, *yao tong* (腰 痛). The accompanying symptoms determine if it is from an emptiness of *yin,* an emptiness of *yang,* a fault in the drawing down of the *qi* by the kidneys, or an overflowing of water through emptiness of the kidneys.

2. Spermatorrhoea, *yi jing* (遺 精), from multiple causes, such as the breaking of communication between the heart and kidneys.

3. Impotence, *yang wei* (陽 痿).

4. Frequent, clear urine; dribbling drop by drop after urination.

5. Deafness, *er long* (耳 聾), and buzzing in the ears, *er ming* (耳 鳴).

6. Superficial oedema, *fu zhong* (浮 腫).

7. Urgent dyspnoea, *chuan* (喘), chronic, with more noticeable difficulty on inspiration.

8. Painful urination, haematuria, polyuria, dysuria.

PRINCIPAL PATTERNS

1. Emptiness of Kidney *yang, shen yang xu* (腎 陽 虛)

Emptiness and decline of the *yang* of the kidneys, *shen yang xu* (腎 陽 虛).

The kidney *qi* no longer ensures firmness, *shen qi bu gu* (腎 氣 不 固).

The kidney no longer draws the *qi* down into the depths, *shen bu na qi* (腎 不 納 氣).

Through emptiness of the kidneys, the water overflows, *shen xu shui fa* (腎 虛 水 泛).

2. Emptiness of kidney *yin, shen yin xu* (腎 陰 虛)

3. Through emptiness of kidney *yin*, the *yang* is too strong, *shen yin xu yang kang* (腎 陰 虛 陽 亢)

INDEX

INDEX